EASY OMT

EASY OMT

A Photo Reference Guide
for
Manual Medical Care

**Step-by-Step Instructions
With Over 300 Photos
of Manual Treatments**

Includes:
Cervicals, Thoracics, Ribs, Lumbars,
Pelvis, Sacrum and Extremities

Written by W. H. Howard, III
Class of 1995
Kirksville College of Osteopathic Medicine

Library of Congress Cataloging-in-Publication Data

Howard, W. H., III

    Easy OMT: a photo-reference guide to manual medical care / by W. H. Howard, III

    p. cm.

    Includes index.

    ISBN 0-9636688-0-3

    92-094309 CIP

Printed in the USA

Published by:

ROB WEAVER, M.B.A.

SPECIALTY PUBLISHING ◆ MARKETING CONSULTING

Street Address: 1009B Mockingbird Lane / Mailing Address: P.O. Box 1176
Siloam Springs, AR 72761

501-524-8400

*With all my love, I dedicate this
book to my wonderful family—
Vicki, Willie, and Chloe.*

Table of Contents

FOREWORD ix
PREFACE..xi
ACKNOWLEDGEMENTS xii
INTRODUCTION xv
HELPFUL HINTS xvii
TREATMENTS
    OA Joint 1
    AA Joint 17
    Typical Cervical C2-C6 21
    Upper Thoracic C7-T3...39
    Lower Thoracic T4-T10 59
    Typical Ribs 2-10 83
    Atypical Ribs 11, 12 103
    Atypical Rib 1 107
    Lumbar T11-L5...117
    Pelvis 139
    Sacrum 165
    Clavicle 195
    Glenohumeral Joint 203
    Ulna 215
    Radius 223
    Wrist 229
    Intercarpal Articulations......................................241
    Carpal Metacarpal Articulation 243
    Metacarpal Phalangeal Articulation.......................245
    Interphalangeal Articulation..................................247
    Hip 249
    Thigh 261
    Knee 263
    Fibula 275
    Ankle 281
    Foot 285
INDEX...299

Foreword

A review of the book, <u>Easy OMT</u>, by Bill Howard, finds it to be as easy to use as counting to 1, 2, 3. Its representative black and white photographs are crisp and clear; and the descriptions are numbered, logical, and to the point.

<u>Easy OMT</u> allows the student or physician to quickly obtain visual and written recall of osteopathic manipulative techniques available for any body region. The book is an excellent refresher of osteopathic treatments as outlined in the <u>Kimberly Manual of Manipulation</u> and supplies the very basic instructions for the execution of each one.

<u>Easy OMT</u> is designed to be useful to a student or physician who needs recall of various valuable techniques and is familiar with the fine points of how to make them effective.

Bill Howard is a student at the Kirksville College of Osteopathic Medicine. He understands student needs which parallel the needs and requirements of a busy general practitioner. I am pleased that Mr. Howard decided to produce this text. Such a work has been needed for a long time and will make a wonderful reference for the professional library of any osteopathic student or physician.

William A. Kuchera, D.O., F.A.A.O.

Preface

During my first year at Kirksville College of Osteopathic Medicine (KCOM), I went through the typical pre-practical paranoia, just like everyone else. In those last few practice hours just before our exam, the OTM lab was alive with students arguing about how a specific technique should be set up, or trying to remember how another treatment should be done. Everyone was frantically trying to leaf through our techniques manual only to discover the detailed, typewritten explanations too time-consuming to wade through.

After surviving three or four practicals, and going through the cram sessions each time, I felt there had to be a way to reduce the anxiousness and make these cram sessions more productive. While I was practicing techniques for the last practical of my first year, the idea struck me— a photo-illustrated, step-by-step book of all the techniques! This would be exactly what every student could use to help quickly answer questions about treatments.

The next day, after my practical, I went to the bookstore to look for such a book. To my amazement, not a single book existed with photos showing treatment set-ups and activating forces for OMT. The bookstore manager told me there was a great demand for such a book, and that many students had asked for one.

Wow! What an opportunity! If I could write such a book, it could be a very useful tool for students, residents and practicing physicians to review treatment techniques for specific diagnoses.

I asked a few classmates what they thought of my idea. They responded positively. The more I thought about it, the more excited I got! With my background in photography, I'd have no problem photographing a treatment set-up in proper sequence and then writing a little text to correspond to the specific hand placement and activation forces.

So, after several months of writing, shooting five-to-six-hundred photographs, many calls to the editor, about 20 proofreadings, and a few other hurdles, **EASY OMT** is now ready for use by anyone who needs a quick, easy-to-use, reference guide for osteopathic manipulative treatments.

If you have comments or suggestions about this book, both what you like about it or ways it can be improved, please write to me, Bill Howard, at: c/o Rob Weaver, P.O. Box 1176, Siloam Springs, Arkansas, 72761.

W. (Bill) H. Howard, III

Acknowledgments

I would like to acknowledge those who stood behind me and encouraged me, as well as helped me write this text. Many thanks to:

God in heaven for instilling in me the idea to write this text.

My wife for believing in me.

Rob and Holly Weaver for research, inputting, and editing.

Dr. Bill Kuchera for writing the foreword and technical editing.

Jay Howard for modeling.

Dana Nelson Howard for assisting in photography.

This book is designed as a quick reference guide for Osteopathic Manipulative Treatments for any area of the body. It assumes the user has medical school training in anatomy and Osteopathic Theory and Manipulation.

Organization and Design of Book

The book begins at the superior parts of the human anatomy and ends with the inferior parts. The page-layout, typefaces and overall design were planned for simple use. Please see the diagram below.

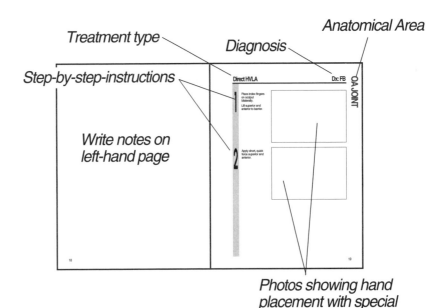

Treatment type

Diagnosis

Anatomical Area

Step-by-step-instructions

Write notes on left-hand page

Photos showing hand placement with special arrows denoting motion

Arrows on the photos represent direction of activating forces necessary to complete the treatment. Arrows depicting **Operator Movement** or **Patient Movement** are designed as shown below.

Operator Movement: Black outline with white inside

Patient Movement: Black outline with black stripes

Arrows with bar: Indicates hold position

1. Definition of Somatic Dysfunction:

Impaired or altered function of the soma, including skeletal, arthroidal, and myofacial structures and related vascular, lymphatic and neural elements.

2. All Treatments:

In any treatment (direct or indirect), patient respiration is usually of great benefit because it helps to flatten out or accentuate spinal curves and relaxes the patient.

Any non-neutral somatic dysfunction needs to be taken care of before a neutral somatic dysfunction is attempted.

3. Indirect Treatments:

When performing indirect treatments, note whether inhalation or exhalation frees the segment with somatic dysfunction most. Then, have the patient hold their breath at that point.

In all indirect treatments, hold segment with somatic dysfunction in "floating" position until a release is felt.

4. Ribs:

When treating ribs (mainly upper ribs), turn patient's head away from side being treated. This helps to free up the costotransverse articulation.

Direct HVLA

1

Place index fingers on occiput bilaterally.

Lift superior and anterior to barrier.

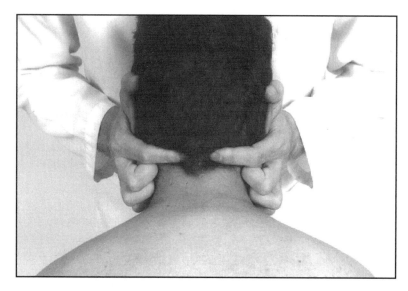

2

Apply short, quick force superior and anterior.

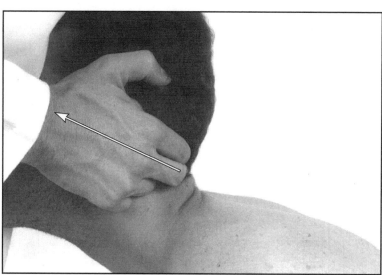

Notes

1

Use thumb and index finger to support C-1 bilaterally.

Let head backward-bend to table.

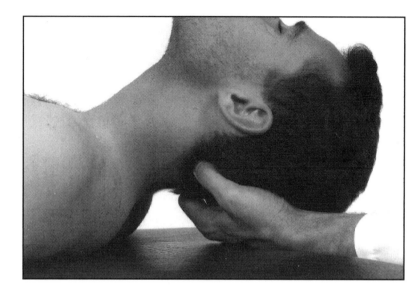

2

Ask patient to lift head against your equally applied force, then relax.

Backward-bend to new barrier again and repeat three to four times.

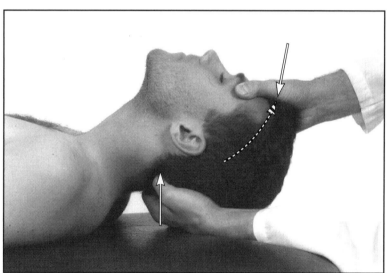

Notes

1 Monitor OA joint with index fingers bilaterally.

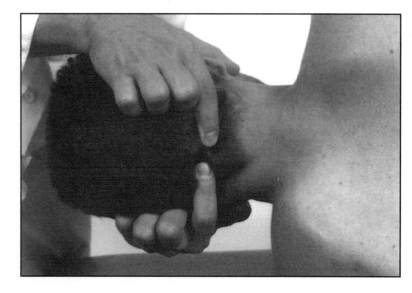

2 Lift head to point of disengaging restrictive barrier.

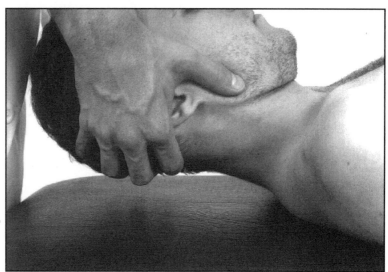

Notes

Direct ME Dx: BB

1

Hold spinous process of C-2 with thumb and index finger of one hand.

With other hand, hold occiput with thumb and index finger.

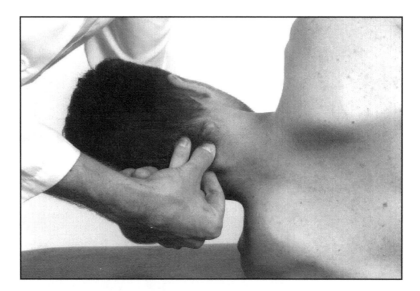

2

Ask patient to place chin on chest.

Hold C-2 firmly while pulling cephlad and anterior on occiput, then relax.

Forward-bend to new barrier again and repeat three to four times.

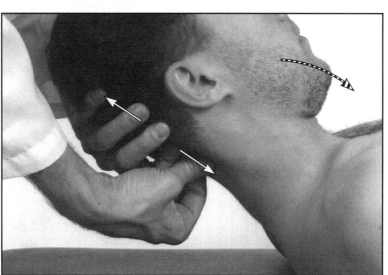

Notes

1

Support head in hands.

Monitor OA joint with index fingers bilaterally.

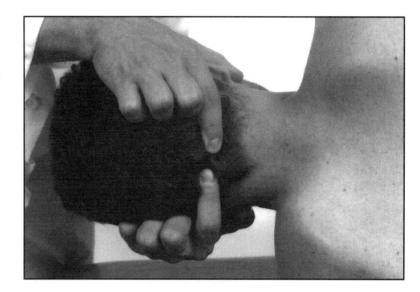

2

Backward-bend patient's head to point of disengaging restrictive barrier.

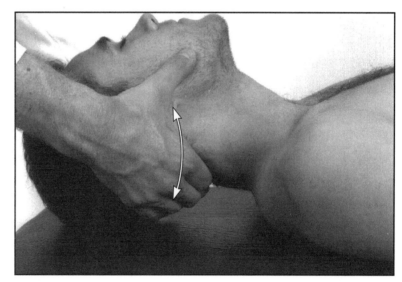

Notes

1 Place index fingers on inferior portion of left occiput just above OA joint.

Side-bend head to left.

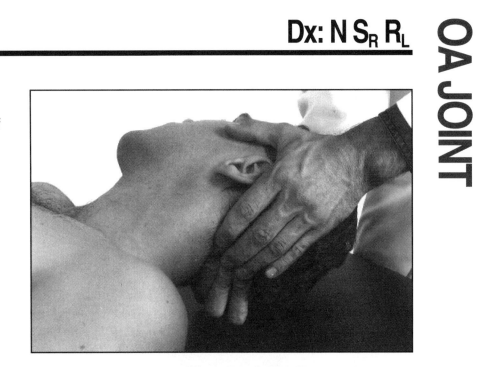

2 Rotate head right to barrier.

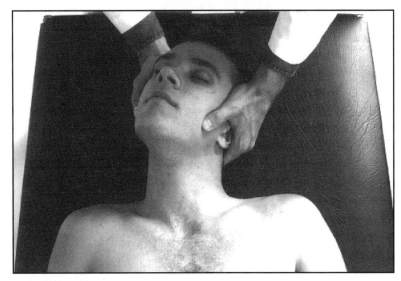

3 Forward-bend or backward-bend to localize.

Apply short, quick thrust towards patient's *right eye*.

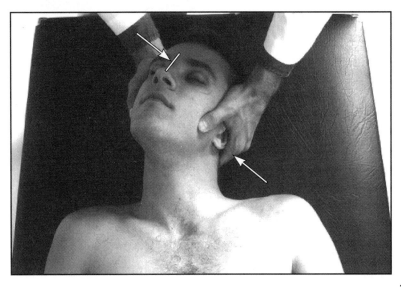

Notes

Direct ME

1 Monitor OA joint with index fingers.

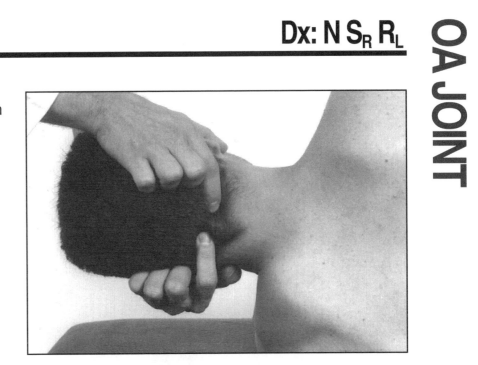

2 Side-bend head left and rotate right to barrier.

Forward-bend or backward-bend to localize.

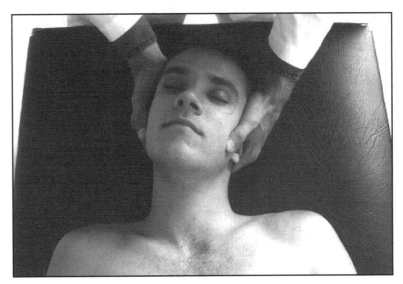

3 Ask patient to look left and rotate head left against your equally applied force, then relax.

Side-bend and rotate to new barrier again and repeat three to four times.

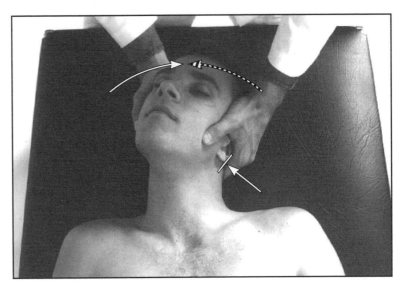

Notes

1 Monitor OA joint with index fingers.

Side-bend right and

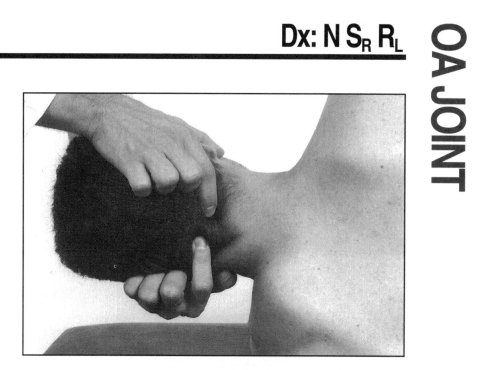

2 rotate left to point of disengaging restrictive barrier.

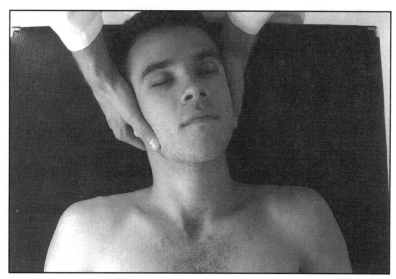

Notes

AA JOINT

1

Place both index fingers on atlas bilaterally.

Support head in hands.

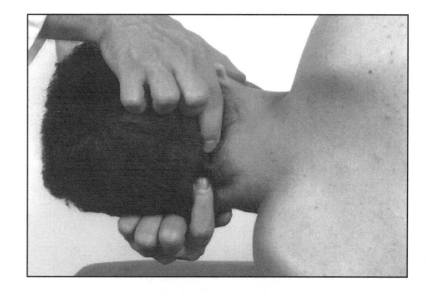

2

Rotate patient's head left to barrier.

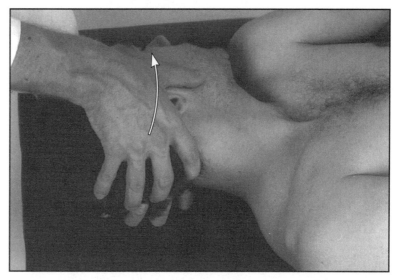

3

Ask patient to rotate head to right against your equally applied force, then relax.

Rotate to new barrier again and repeat three to four times.

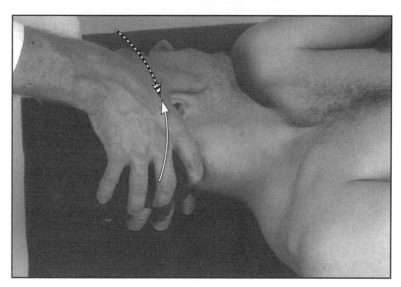

Notes

1 Place left index finger on left lateral mass of C-1.

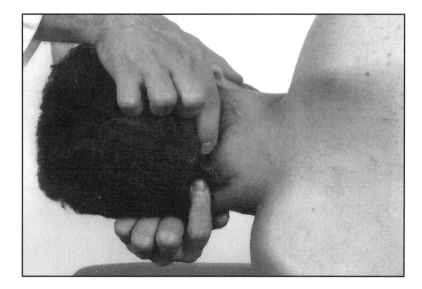

2 Support head with hands and rotate right to point of disengaging restrictive barrier.

(Lifting or lowering head may be necessary, as well as pressure from left index finger.)

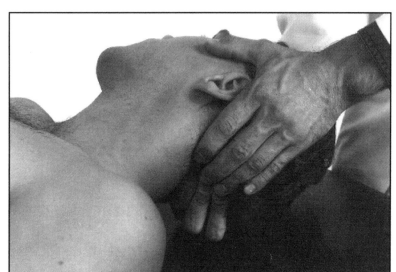

Notes

TYPICAL CERVICAL C2-C6

1 Place index fingers at segment with somatic dysfunction.

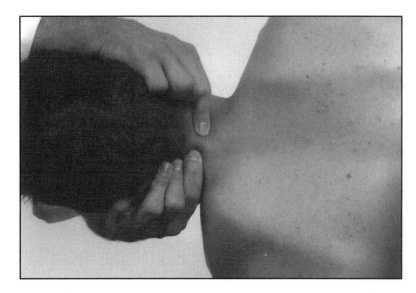

2 Lift superior and anterior to barrier.

Apply short, quick thrust superior and anterior.

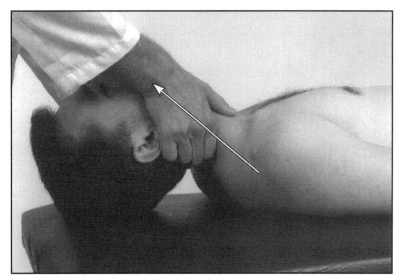

Notes

Direct ME

1 Place thumb and index finger bilaterally on articular pillars at segment with somatic dysfunction.

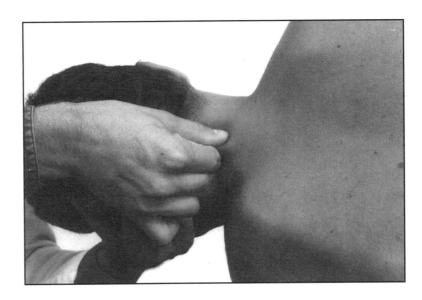

2 Lift superior and anterior to barrier.

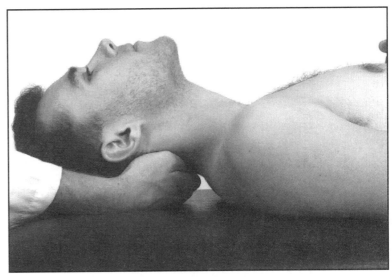

3 Ask patient to lift head against your equally applied force, then relax.

Lift to new barrier again and repeat three to four times.

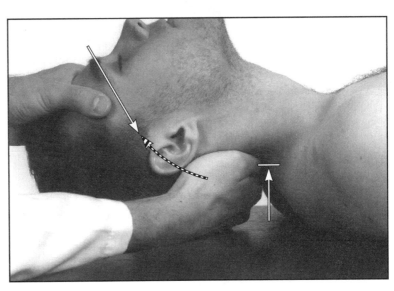

Notes

Indirect

1 Place thumb and index finger on spinous process of segment with somatic dysfunction.

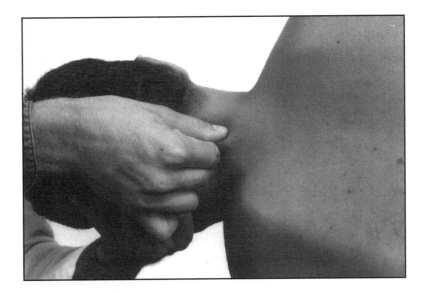

2 Disengage restrictive barrier by increasing or decreasing pressure on segment with somatic dysfunction.

Hold in disengaged position until release is felt.

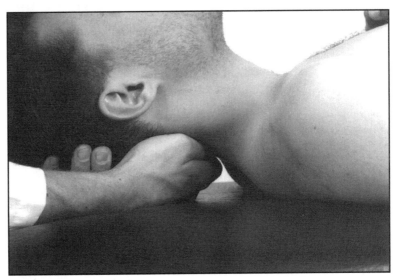

TYPICAL CERVICAL C2-C6

Notes

TYPICAL CERVICAL C2-C6

1

Use thumb and index finger to hold segment *below* somatic dysfunction on posterior vertebral arches.

Support patient's head.

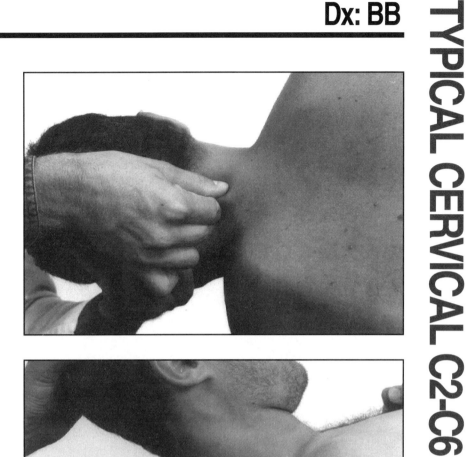

2

Lift head to barrier.

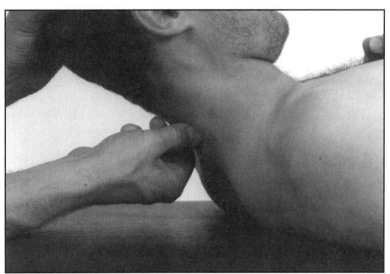

3

Ask patient to press head against your equally applied force, then relax.

Lift to new barrier again and repeat three to four times.

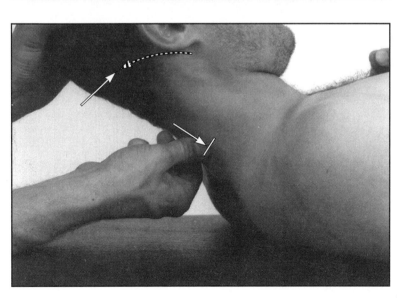

Notes

1 Place index fingers bilaterally on articular pillars.

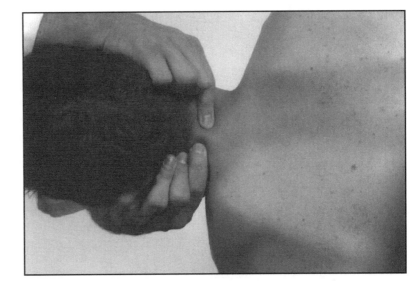

2 Press anterior to point of disengaging restrictive barrier of segment with somatic dysfunction.

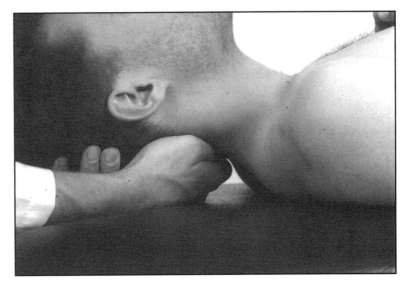

Notes

Direct HVLA (Side-bending)

Dx: N S$_R$ R$_R$

1 Place lateral aspect of left index finger slightly below point of fullness.

Side-bend left down to barrier.

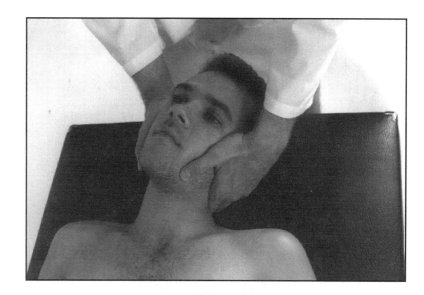

2 Rotate right to lock out upper segments.

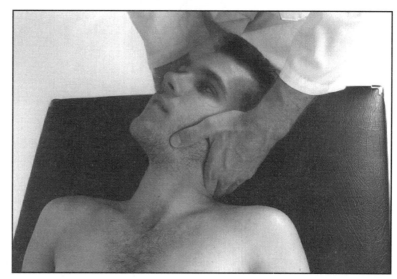

3 Apply short, quick thrust toward patient's *right* nipple.

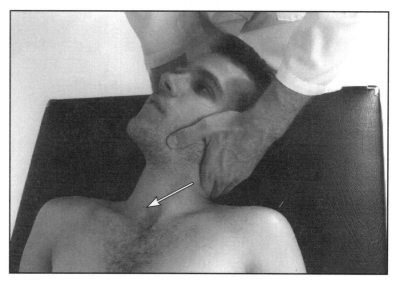

Notes

Direct ME

Dx: N S$_R$ R$_R$

1 Place lateral aspect of left index finger slightly below point of fullness.

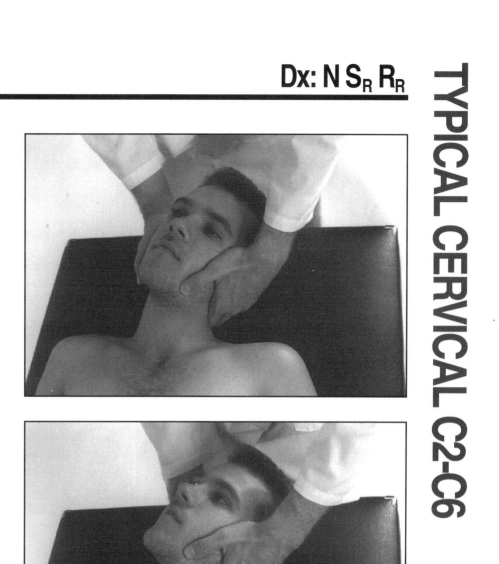

2 Side-bend and rotate left down to barrier.

3 Ask patient to side-bend head to right against your equally applied force, then relax.

Side-bend patient's head to new barrier again and repeat three to four times.

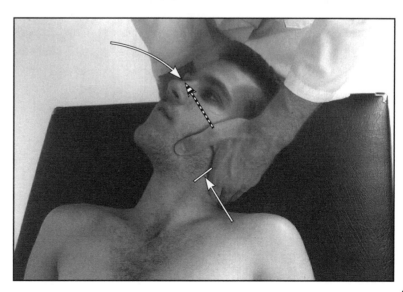

Notes

Indirect

Dx: N S_R R_R

1 Side-bend *right* and rotate *right* until disengaging restrictive barrier.

(Some pressure on left articular pillar at segment with somatic dysfunction may be helpful.)

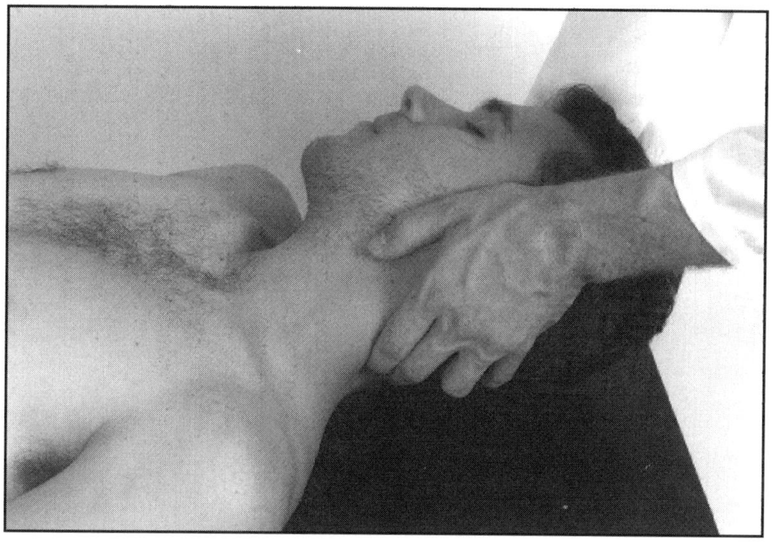

Notes

TYPICAL CERVICAL C2-C6

1

This can be corrected using procedures for **Diagnosis: N S_R R_R**, shown on pages 31 to 35.

Be sure to check forward-bending component and treat first if necessary.

Please see pages 31 to 35.

Notes

Direct Springing

1 Place middle, ring and index fingers on upper sternal body.

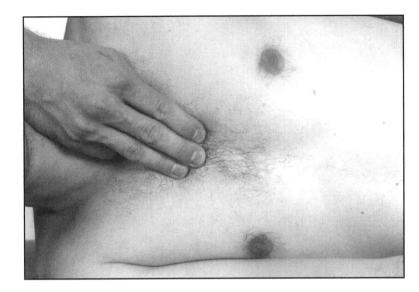

2 Place heel of opposite hand on spinous process of segment(s) with somatic dysfunction.

Spring anterior and inferior.

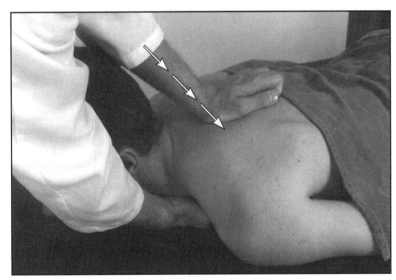

Notes

Direct Springing

1

Ask patient to sit with arms crossed (photo).

Spring caudal and anterior while patient relaxes on operator.

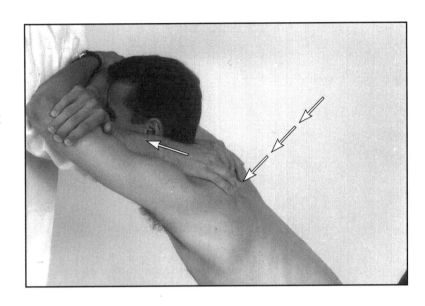

Notes

1 Monitor worst segment with index finger of both hands.

Lift patient's head to point of disengaging restrictive barrier of segment with somatic dysfunction.

Hold in disengaged position until release is felt.

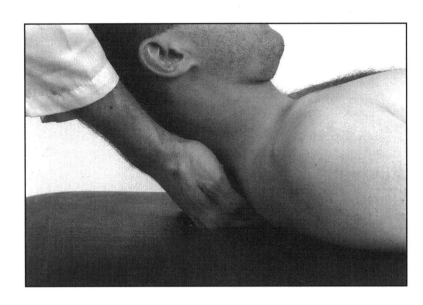

UPPER THORACIC C7-T3

Notes

Direct HVLA

1 Place hand caudal to segment with somatic dysfunction.

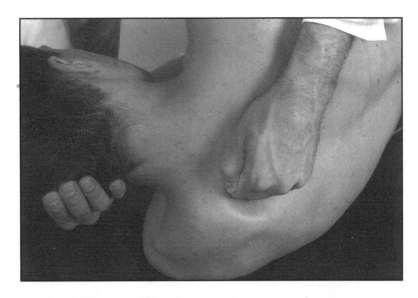

2 Maintain patient's head in *forward-bending* position and localize to barrier of segment with somatic dysfunction.

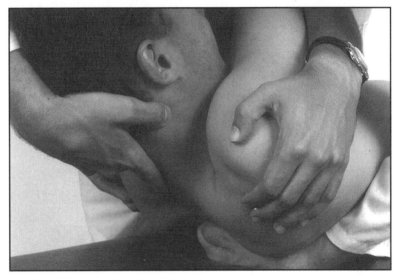

3 Apply short, quick force in posterior superior *(45 degrees)* direction.

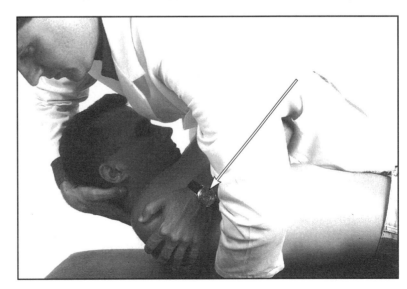

Notes

UPPER THORACIC C7-T3

1 Hold segment caudal to somatic dysfunction in fixed position.

Forward-bend patient's head until localized at barrier.

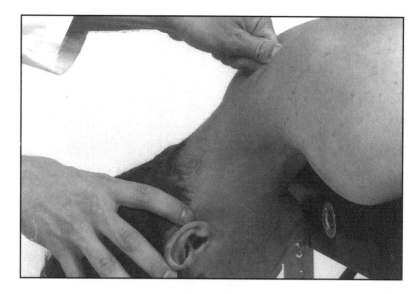

2 Ask patient to backward-bend head against your equally applied force, then relax.

Lower to new barrier again and repeat three to four times.

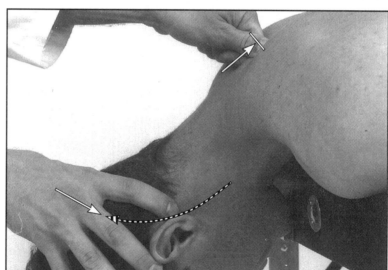

Notes

1 Place index finger on segment with somatic dysfunction and press anterior to point of disengaging restrictive barrier of segment with somatic dysfunction.

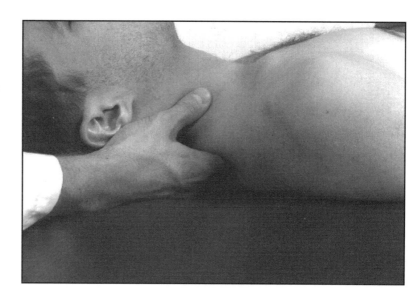

Notes

Direct HVLA

$$Dx: N\ S_R\ R_L$$

1 Using thumb, monitor left transverse process of segment with somatic dysfunction.

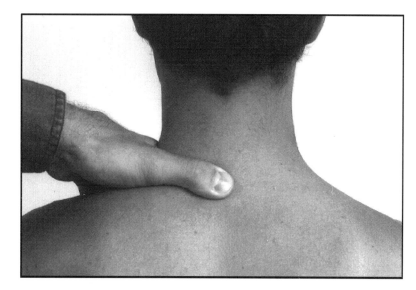

2 Ask patient to lean to the right and relax on your knee.

Apply short, quick force with your left hand at 45 degrees medial and inferior.

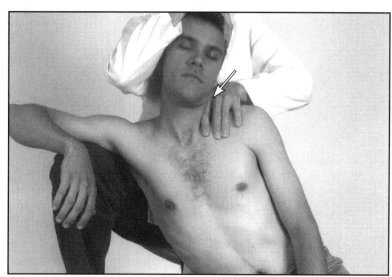

Notes

Direct ME

1

Translate to right down to segment with somatic dysfunction.

Ask patient to sit erect.

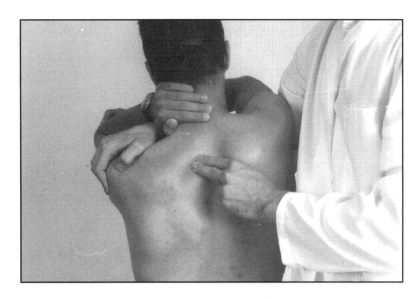

2

Rotate to *right* down to segment with somatic dysfunction.

While applying anterior force on the left transverse process, ask patient to rotate left against your equally applied force, then relax.

Translate and rotate to new barrier again and repeat three to four times.

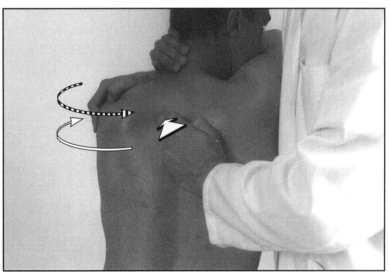

Notes

Dx: N S$_R$ R$_L$

1

Place index finger on right transverse process.

Raise, lower, and/or side-bend head to disengage restrictive barrier of segment with somatic dysfunction.

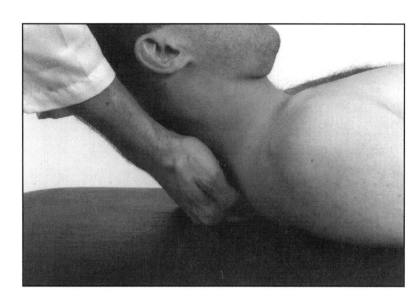

Notes

1

This can be corrected using procedures for **Diagnosis: BB**.

Please see pages 45 to 49.

Notes

Direct HVLA

1

Place heel of hand on spinous process of segment with somatic dysfunction.

Apply short, quick thrust directly anterior.

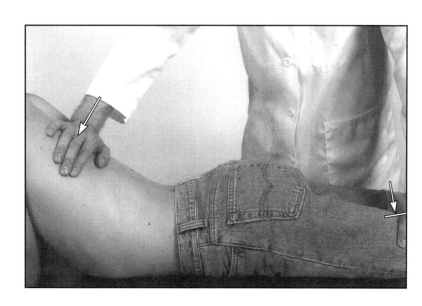

Notes

Direct HVLA

LOWER THORACIC T4-T10

1 Place hands as shown in photo.

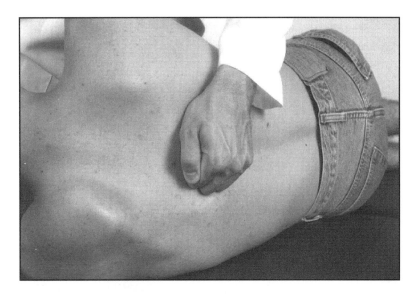

2 Localize directly over your hand while maintaining general forward-bending position.

Apply short, quick thrust toward table.

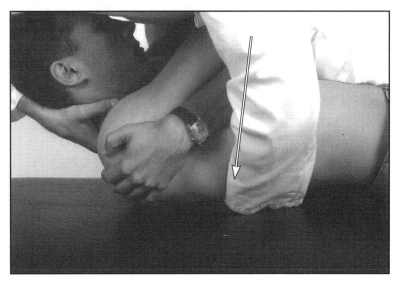

Notes

1 Spring caudal and anterior at area with somatic dysfunction while patient relaxes weight on your arms.

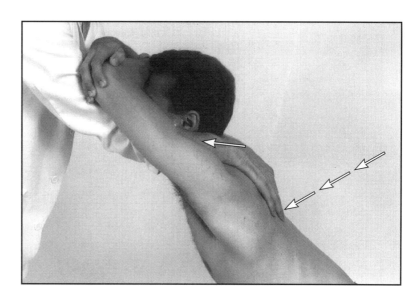

LOWER THORACIC T4-T10

Notes

Direct HVLA

1 Place hand caudal to segment with somatic dysfunction.

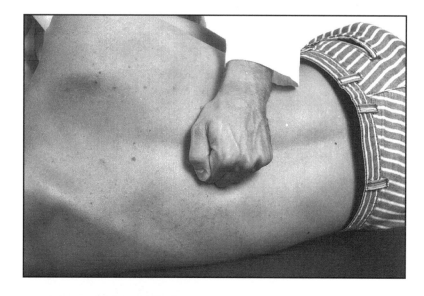

2 Maintain patient's head in *forward-bending* position and localize to barrier of segment with somatic dysfunction.

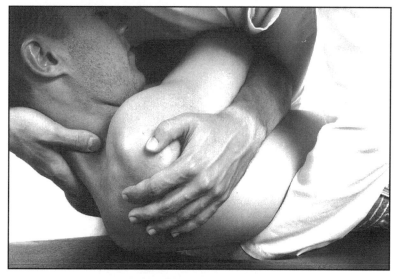

3 Apply short, quick force at 45 degrees posterior and superior.

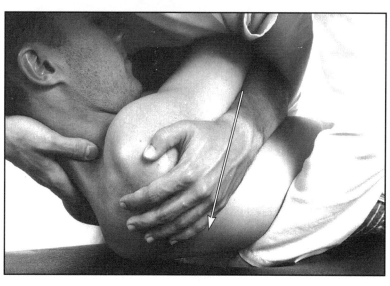

Notes

1

Hold segment below somatic dysfunction.

Ask patient to arch back at segment. (Crossing patient's arms helps to arch back).

Ask patient to sit erect against your equally applied force, then relax.

Ask patient to arch back to new barrier again and repeat three to four times.

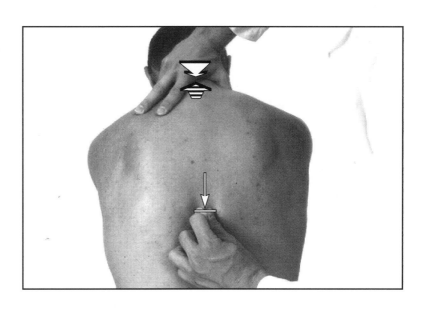

Notes

1 Place fingers on segment with somatic dysfunction.

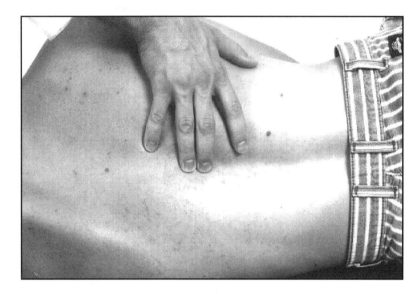

2 Press anterior to point of disengaging restrictive barrier.

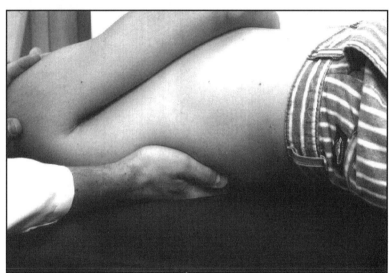

LOWER THORACIC T4-T10

Notes

Direct HVLA

Dx: N S$_L$ R$_R$

LOWER THORACIC T4-T10

1 Open hand and place thenar eminence on right transverse process of segment with somatic dysfunction.

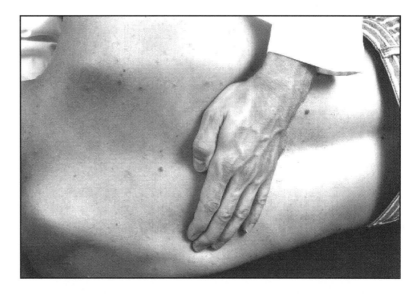

2 Side-bend right (away from operator).

Apply short, quick force at 90 degrees to table (posterior).

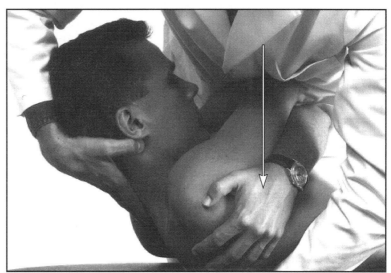

Notes

Direct ME

Dx: N S$_L$ R$_R$

1 With thumb, contact spinous process of segment with somatic dysfunction and push to induce rotation left.

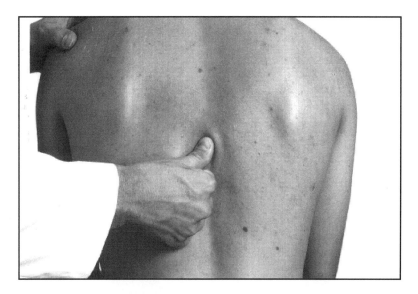

2 Side-bend patient right to barrier.

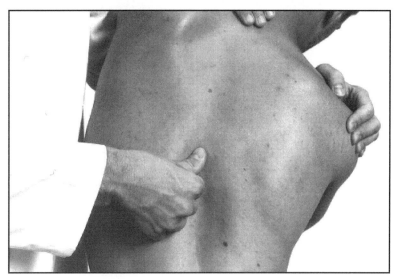

3 Ask patient to side-bend against your equally applied force, then relax.

Side-bend patient to new barrier again and repeat three to four times.

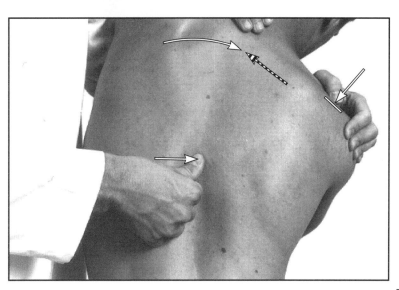

Notes

1

Side-bend patient left.

Place index and/or middle finger on spinous process of segment with somatic dysfunction.

Pull spinous process until restrictive barrier is disengaged.

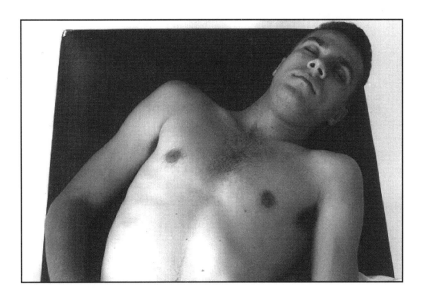

Notes

Direct HVLA

$Dx: NN\ R_R\ S_R$

1 Open hand and place thenar eminence on right transverse process of segment with somatic dysfunction.

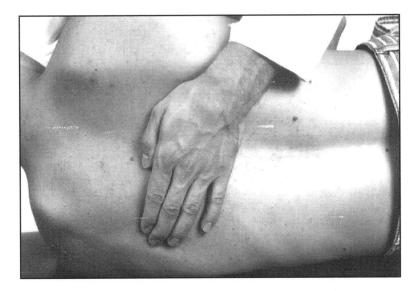

2 Side-bend left (towards operator) while maintaining forward-bending position.

Apply short, quick force at 45 degrees posterior and superior.

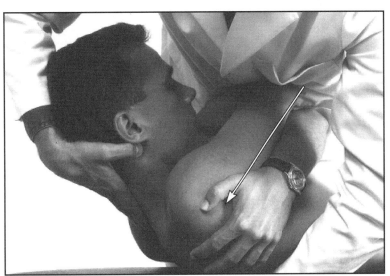

LOWER THORACIC T4-T10

Notes

1 Place thumb on right transverse process.

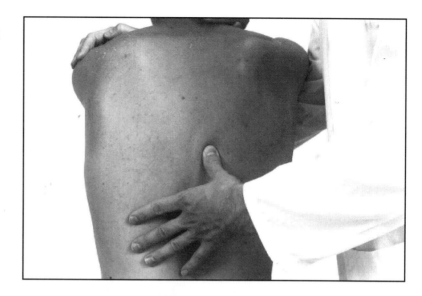

2 Support and side-bend patient left down to barrier.

(Asking patient to sit erect or slump may help localize barrier.)

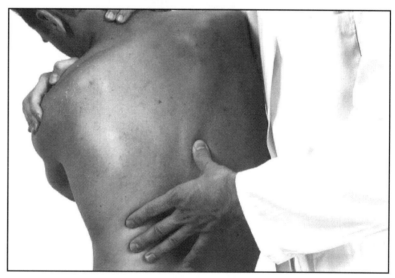

3 Using thumb to apply pressure, ask patient to side-bend right against your equally applied force, then relax.

Side-bend patient to new barrier again and repeat three to four times.

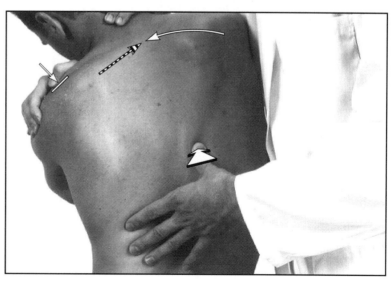

Notes

1 Place index and middle fingers on spinous process of segment with somatic dysfunction.

Side-bend patient right.

Disengage restrictive barrier of segment with somatic dysfunction by applying pressure as needed on spinous process.

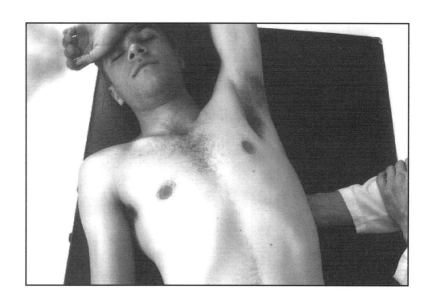

LOWER THORACIC T4-T10

Notes

Direct HVLA

Dx: Inhalation*

*(Pump handle, 2-7, usually in groups)

1 Place heel of hand on angle of rib.

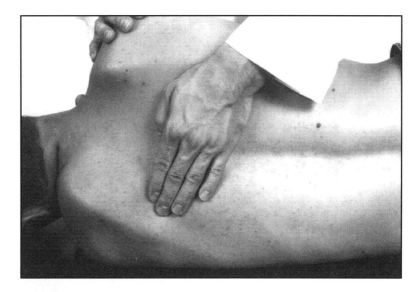

2 Localize over rib with somatic dysfunction, using a short, quick, cephlad force, pivoting around wrist.

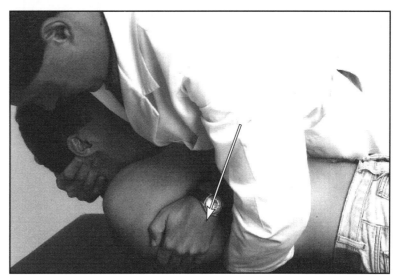

83

Notes

Direct Respiratory

Dx: Inhalation*

*(Pump handle, 2-7, usually in groups)

1

Hold angle of rib with one hand and pull cephlad.

Lift patient to localize rib(s) to be treated.

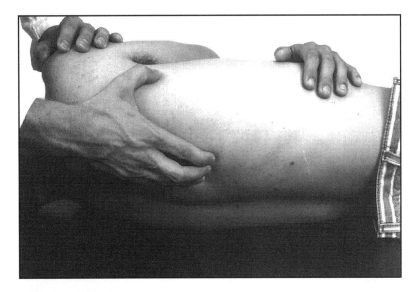

2

Press on anterior aspect of rib being treated as patient exhales.

Repeat two to three times.

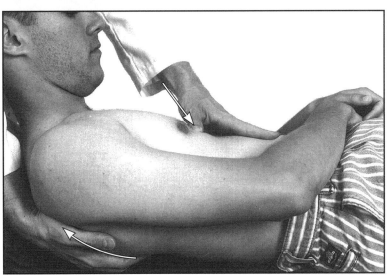

Notes

*(Pump handle, 2-7, usually in groups)

1 Place hands on angle of rib posterior, and in intercostal spaces anterior.

Move rib to point of disengaging restrictive barrier and hold until release is felt.

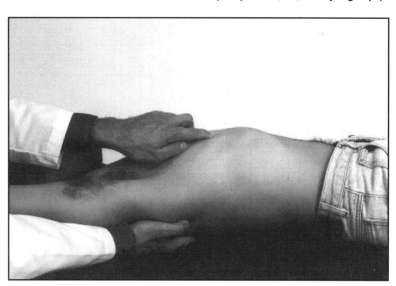

Notes

*(Bucket Handle: Ribs 4-10)

1 Contact angle of rib with somatic dysfunction with one hand.

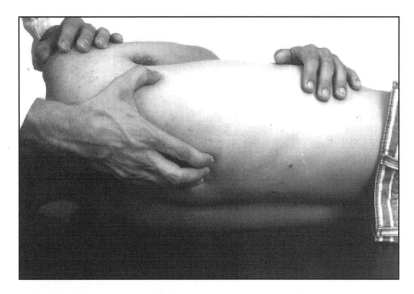

2 Rest patient's head on your knee.

Forward-bend and side-bend patient towards side with somatic dysfunction to localize barrier.

Press inferior with opposite hand as shown.

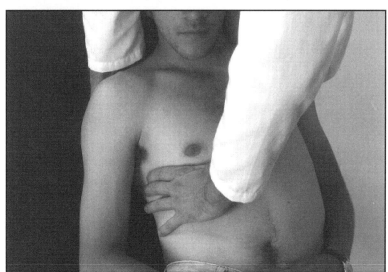

3 Ask patient to side-bend away against your equally applied force, then relax.

Forward-bend and side-bend patient to new barrier again and repeat three to four times.

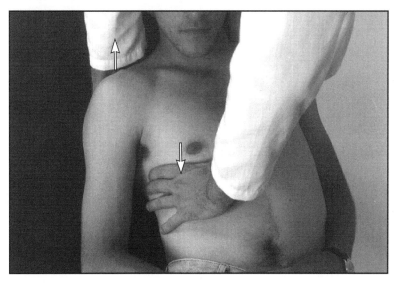

Notes

Dx: Inhalation*

*(Bucket Handle: Ribs 4-10)

1

Place hands on angle of rib and on anterior end of rib.

Place thumbs on mid-axillary line of rib.

Press angle and anterior end gently together until restrictive rib/ribs are disengaged.

Hold until release is felt.

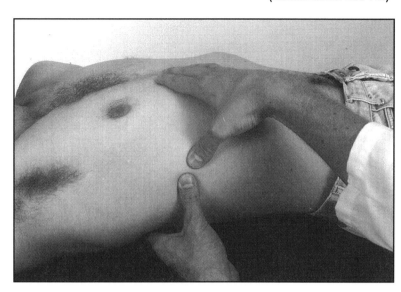

Notes

Direct HVLA

1 Place heel of hand on angle of rib.

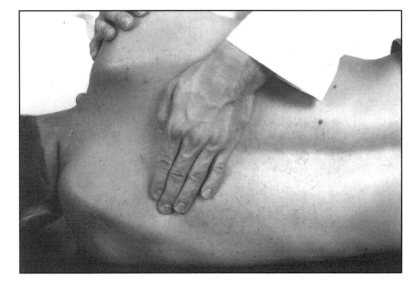

2 Localize over rib with somatic dysfunction, using a short, quick, caudal force, pivoting around wrist.

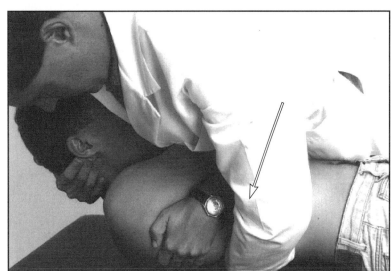

Notes

TYPICAL RIB 2-10

1

Contact angle of rib with somatic dysfunction with middle, ring, and index fingers.

Pull caudal.

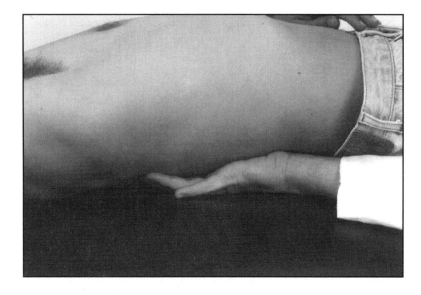

2

Ask patient to raise arm above head.

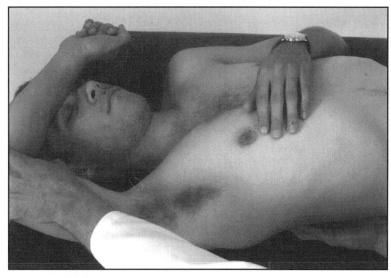

3

While maintaining caudal force on rib angle, ask patient to lower arm against your equally applied force, then relax.

Approach new barrier again and repeat three to four times.

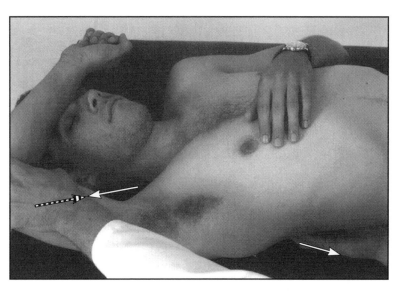

Notes

*(Bucket handle)

1

Contact angle of dysfunctional rib with one hand and anterior end with the other.

Thumbs should contact rib near mid-axillary line.

Move rib towards point of disengaging restrictive barrier and hold until release is felt.

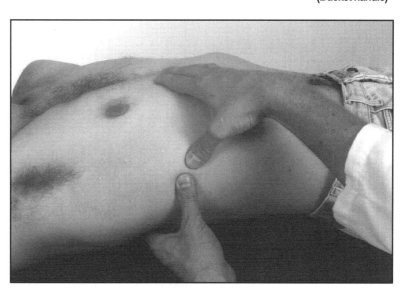

Notes

1 Contact angle of dysfunctional rib with middle, ring, and index fingers.

Pull caudal.

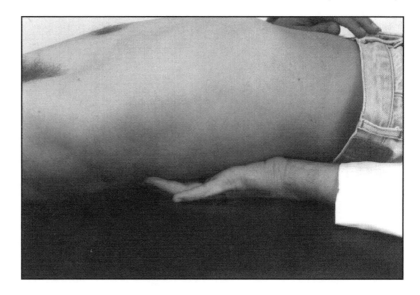

2 Ask patient to raise arm above head.

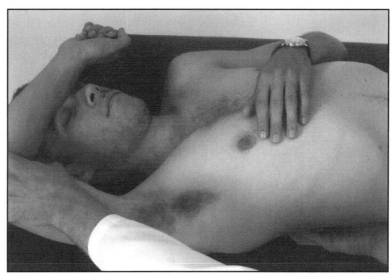

3 While maintaining caudal force on rib angle, ask patient to lower arm down to *side* against your equally applied force, then relax.

Pull rib caudal to new barrier again and repeat three to four times.

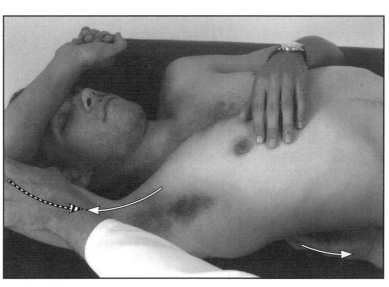

Notes

1

Contact angle of dysfunctional rib with one hand and the anterior end with the other.

Thumbs should contact rib near mid-axillary line.

Move rib towards point of disengaging restrictive barrier and hold until release is felt.

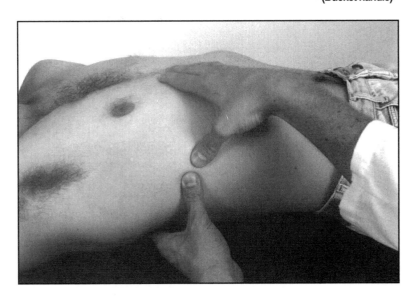

Notes

1

Side-bend patient to opposite side of somatic dysfunction.

Place thumb (fulcrum) on posterior inferior aspect of costotransverse joint.

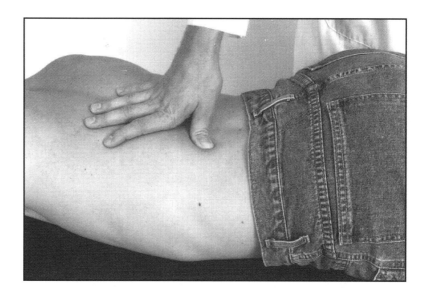

2

By grasping ASIS, raise hip while maintaining superior anterior force on costotransverse joint.

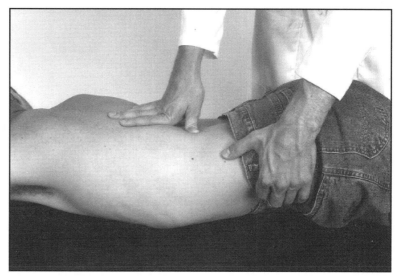

3

Ask patient to press hip down towards table against your equally applied force, then relax.

Approach new barrier again and repeat three to four times.

(Having patient exhale while approaching barrier may be helpful.)

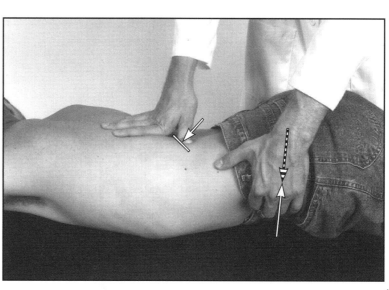

Notes

1 Side-bend patient to opposite side of somatic dysfunction.

Brace shaft of rib with somatic dysfunction with anterolateral portion of thumb.

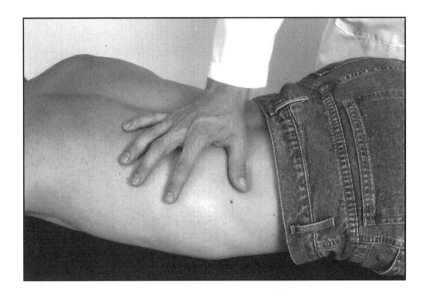

2 By grasping ASIS, raise hip while maintaining superior anterior force on rib shaft.

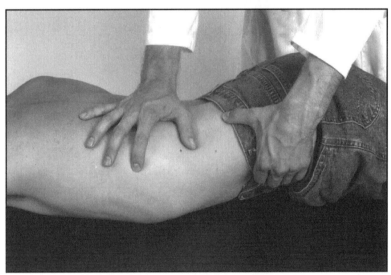

3 Ask patient to press hip down towards table against your equally applied force, then relax.

Approach new barrier again and repeat three to four times.

(Having patient exhale while approaching barrier may be helpful.)

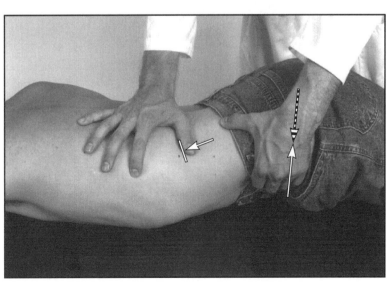

Notes

1 Contact superior and posterior portion of rib 1 (photo).

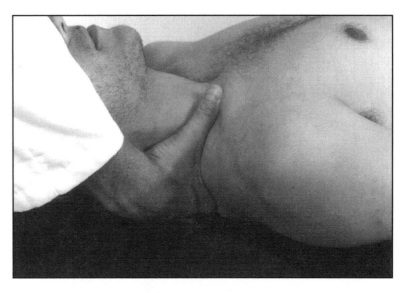

2 Rotate head away and side-bend down to barrier.

(Forward-bending or backward-bending at point of C-7 and T-1 to localize barrier is helpful.)

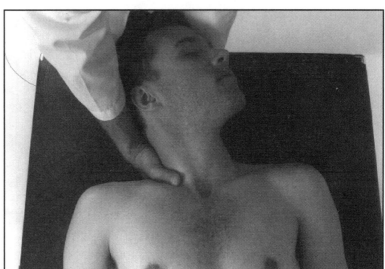

3 Apply short, quick force toward opposite nipple.

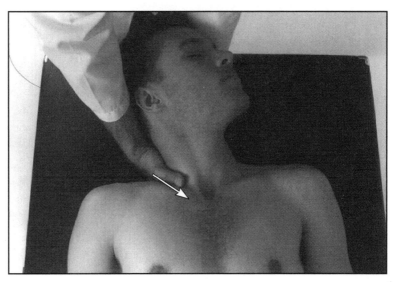

Notes

1 Contact superior and posterior portion of rib 1 (photo).

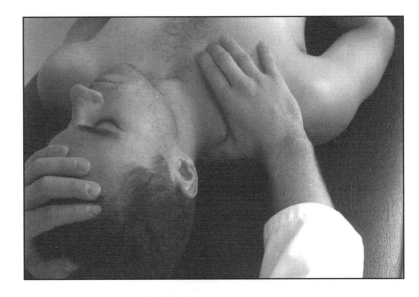

2 Rotate head to opposite side of rib with somatic dysfunction.

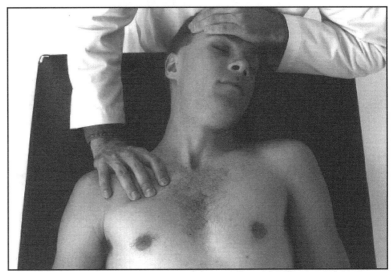

3 Press caudal on rib and shoulder to barrier.

Ask patient to raise head against your equally applied force, then relax.

Press caudal to new barrier again and repeat three to four times.

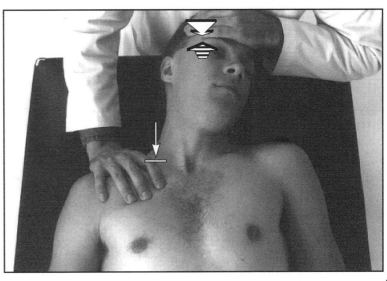

Notes

ATYPICAL RIB 1

1 Place thumb on angle of rib one.

Place index and middle fingers on anterior medial shaft, just superior to the sternoclavicular joint.

Forward- or backward-bending will help to localize barrier.

Lift rib to point of disengaging restrictive barrier and maintain until release is felt.

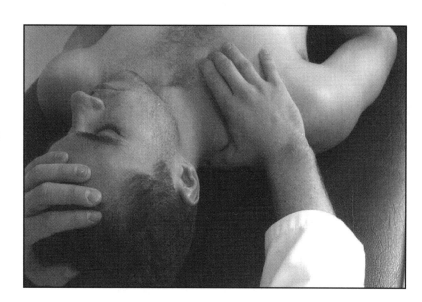

Notes

1 Place middle, ring, and index finger on superior posterior aspect of first rib.

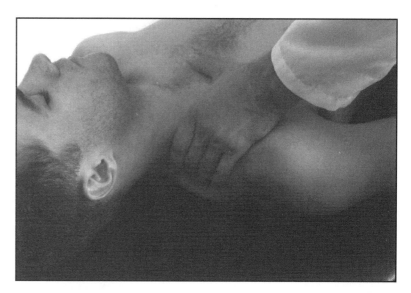

2 Ask patient to raise head against your equally applied force, then relax.

Repeat three to four times.

(Note: force of hand on first rib is anterior, inferior and lateral).

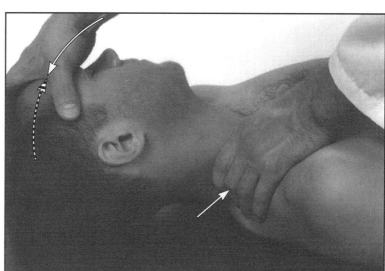

Notes

1

Place thumb on angle of rib one.

Place index and middle fingers on anterior medial shaft.

Depress rib to point of disengaging restrictive barrier and maintain until release is felt.

(Side-bending head towards side with somatic dysfunction may be helpful.)

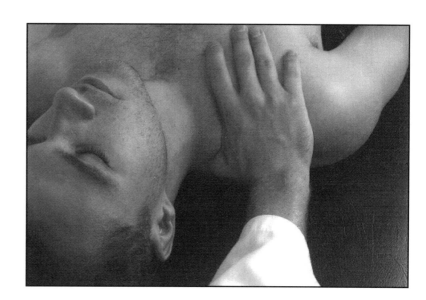

Notes

Direct HVLA

1

Place thenar eminence on spinous process of segment with somatic dysfunction.

Increase pressure until barrier is reached.

Apply short, quick force toward table.

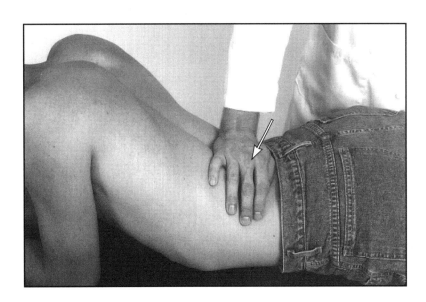

Notes

1 Place thenar eminence on segment with somatic dysfunction.

Backward-bend down to barrier.

Ask patient to forward bend against your equally applied force, then relax.

Backward-bend patient to new barrier again and repeat three to four times.

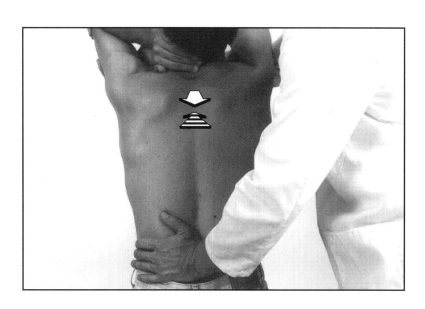

Notes

1

Caution is advised if shoulder problems exist.

Ask patient to place bare buttocks on table (for resistance).

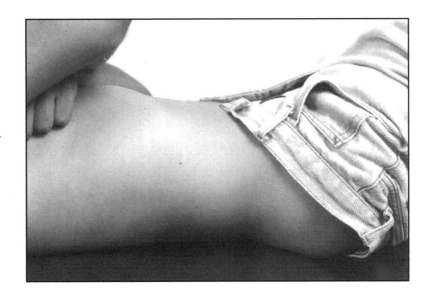

2

Grasp patient's arms and pull until barrier is met.

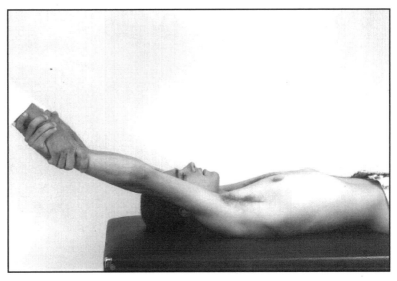

3

Apply short, quick pull on arms.

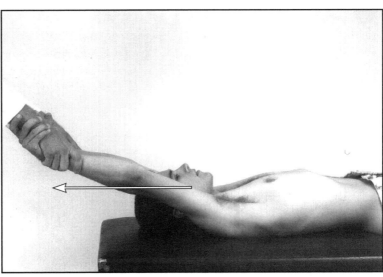

Notes

1 Ask patient to flex knees and raise up to chest.

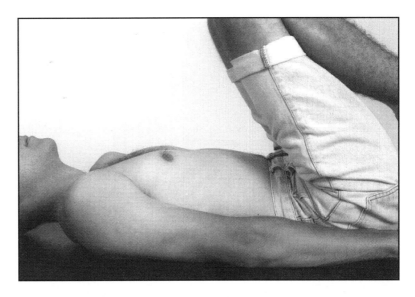

2 Place index and/or middle finger bilaterally on segment with somatic dysfunction.

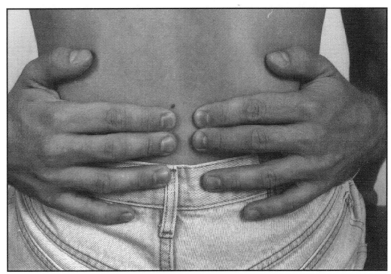

3 Apply pressure on knees to reach barrier.

Ask patient to press knees out against your equally applied force, then relax.

Apply pressure to reach new barrier again and repeat three to four times.

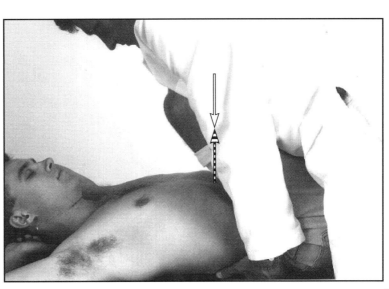

Notes

1 Place index and
middle finger on
spinous process.

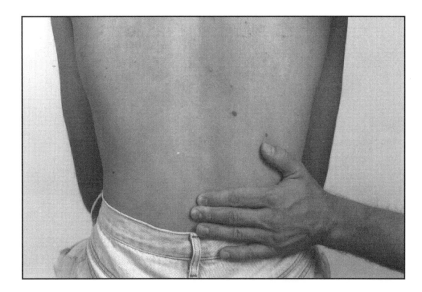

2 Press anterior to
disengage restrictive
barrier of segment
with somatic
dysfunction.

Hold until release is
felt.

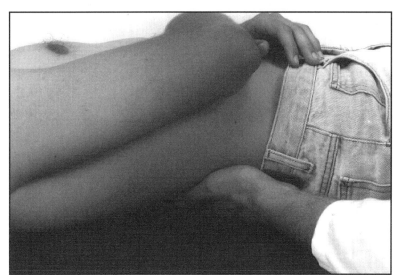

Notes

1 Place index and/or middle fingers on segment with somatic dysfunction to monitor localization.

Flex upper leg to localize barrier and straighten lower leg.

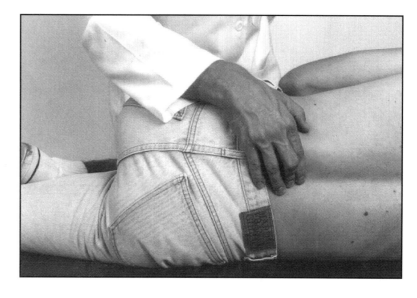

2 Pull lower shoulder cephlad and anterior.

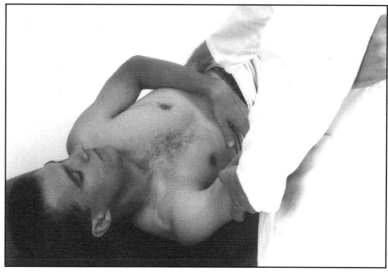

3 Control upper shoulder with one arm.

Place other forearm posterior to greater trochanter and pull until barrier is reached.

Stabilize patient's shoulder while applying short, quick thrust on pelvis anterior, superior and medial.

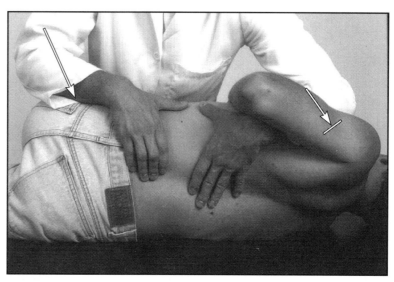

Notes

1 Place index finger on spinous process of segment with somatic dysfunction.

Pull spinous process to rotate segment left.

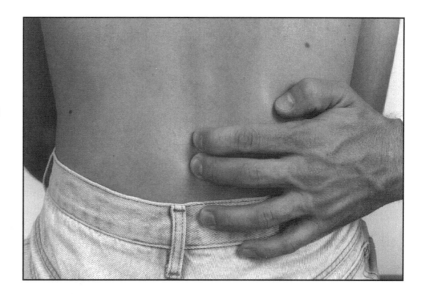

2 Ask patient to flex knees and place them on right side of table.

While continuing to hold pressure on segment with somatic dysfunction, grasp patient's ankle with the other hand.

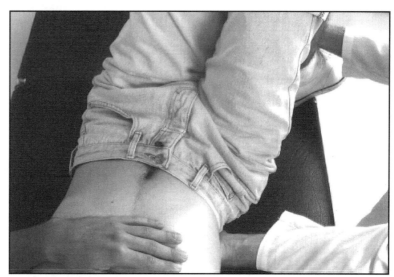

3 Ask patient to move feet to mid-line against your equally applied force, then relax.

Pull spinous process and side-bend patient to new barrier again and repeat three to four times.

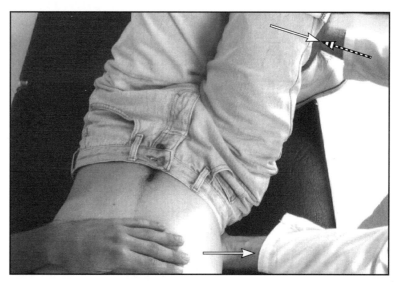

Notes

LUMBAR T11-L5

1

Place index and middle fingers on spinous process of segment with somatic dysfunction.

Translate patient's shoulders to the left to induce slight right side-bending.

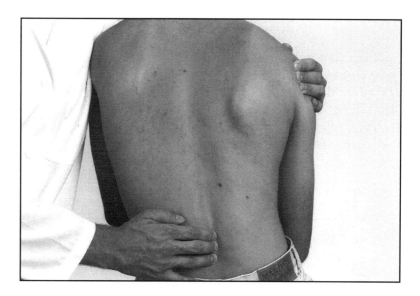

2

Push spinous process to disengage restrictive barrier of segment with somatic dysfunction.

Hold until release is felt.

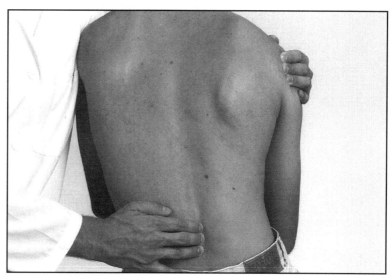

Notes

1 Place heel of hand on right aspect of spinous process of segment with somatic dysfunction.

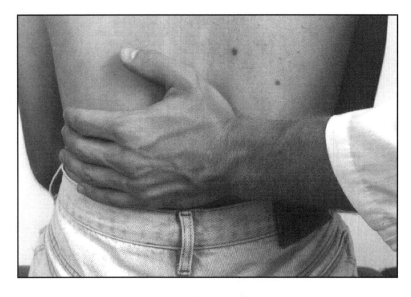

2 Rotate, side-bend and backward-bend patient to localize barrier.

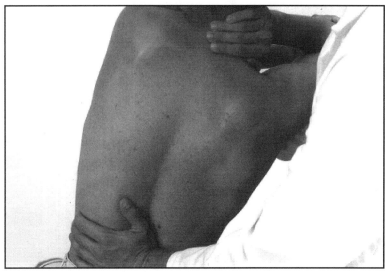

3 Apply short, quick thrust toward patient's opposite hip.

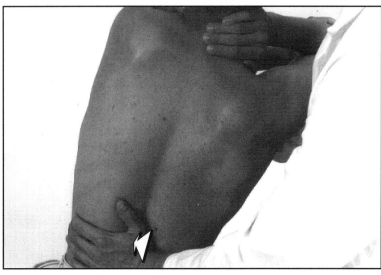

Notes

Dx: NN R_L S_L

1 Place heel of hand on right aspect of spinous process of segment with somatic dysfunction.

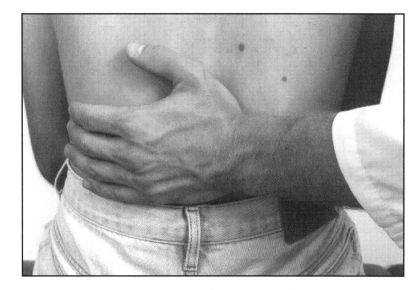

2 Rotate, side-bend and backward-bend patient to localize barrier.

Ask patient to rotate left against your equally applied force, then relax.

Rotate, side-bend and backward-bend to new barrier again and repeat three to four times.

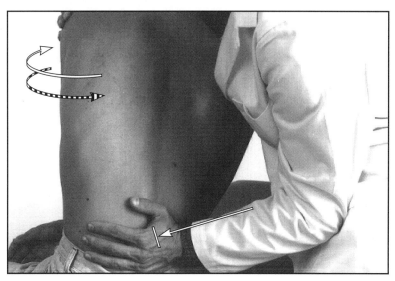

Notes

1 Ask patient to flex knees and place feet flat on table.

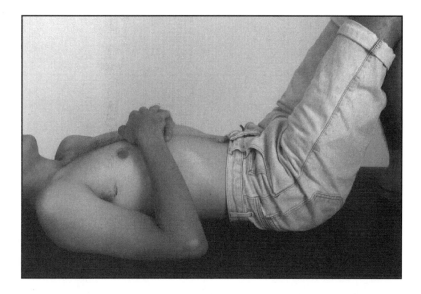

2 Place index and/or middle finger on spinous process and float segment.

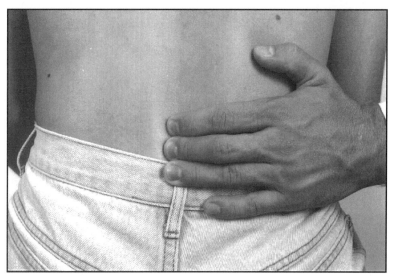

3 Ask patient to side-bend until restrictive barrier of segment with somatic dysfunction is disengaged.

Hold until release is felt.

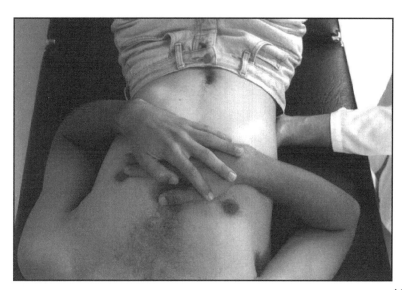

Notes

1

Place hands as shown in photo.

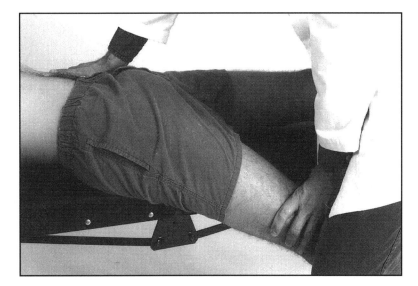

2

Press down on patient's knee to point of ligamentous tension.

Ask patient to raise knee against your equally applied force, then relax.

Press down on knee to new barrier and repeat three to four times.

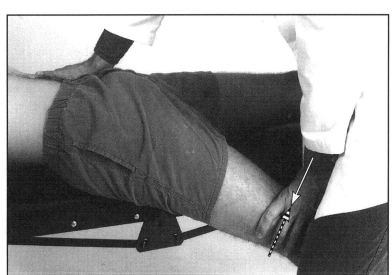

Notes

1

Place thumb and index finger of each hand on pubic body bilaterally.

Move pubes in opposite directions to disengage restrictive barrier.

Hold until release is felt.

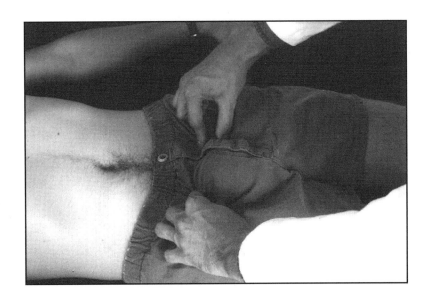

Notes

1 With caudal hand, grasp ischial tuberosity.

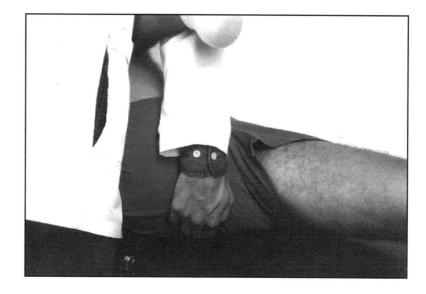

2 Place thenar eminance of cephlad hand against anterior inferior aspect of ASIS.

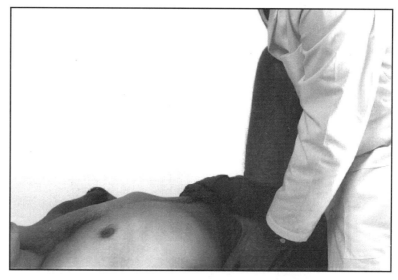

3 Lean on patient's knee to flex and *abduct* the thigh to the point of ligamentous tension.

Ask patient to press knee against your equally applied force, then relax.

Flex and *abduct* thigh to new barrier and repeat three to four times.

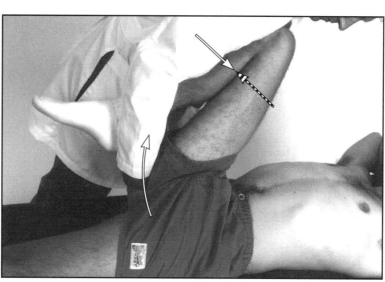

Notes

1

Place thumb and index finger of each hand on pubic body bilaterally.

Move pubes in opposite directions to disengage restrictive barrier.

Hold until release is felt.

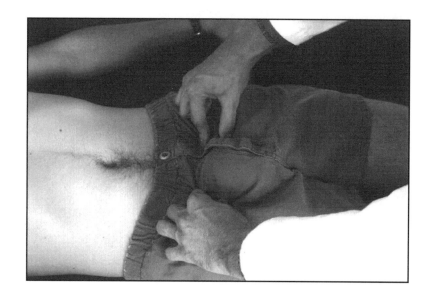

Notes

1

Ask patient to flex knees and hips.

Hold knees together as patient tries to abduct them.

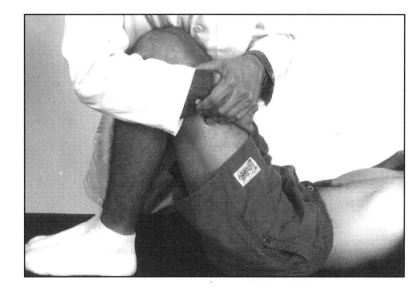

2

Separate patient's knees by placing forearm between.

Ask patient to bring knees together with a fairly strong effort, then relax.

Repeat two to three times.

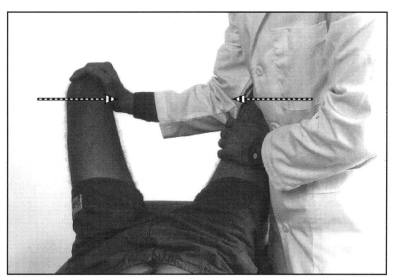

Notes

1 Place heel of hand slightly superior to PSIS.

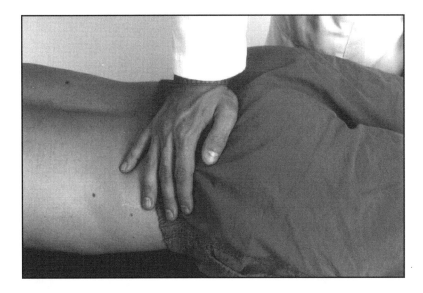

2 Lift patient's leg to point of ligamentous tension.

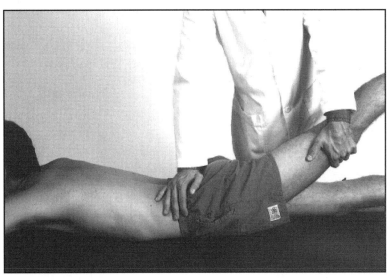

3 Apply short, quick thrust anterior while lifting patient's leg.

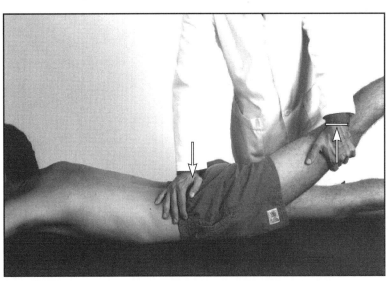

Notes

1 Place heel of hand slightly superior to PSIS.

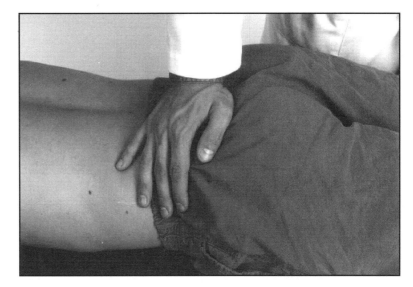

2 Lift patient's leg to point of ligamentous tension.

Ask patient to lower leg towards table against your equally applied force, then relax.

Lift leg to new barrier again and repeat three to four times.

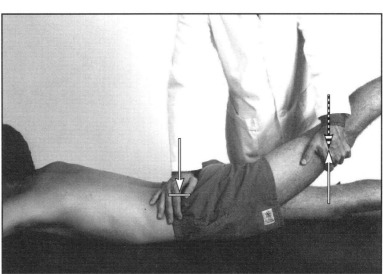

Notes

1

Place hands as
shown in photo.

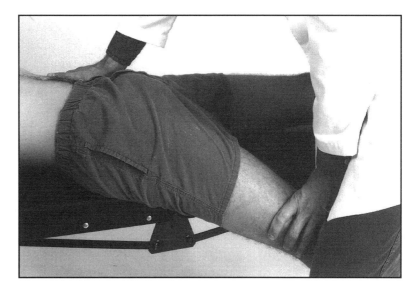

2

Press down on
patient's knee to
point of ligamentous
tension.

Ask patient to raise
knee against your
equally applied
force, then relax.

Press down on knee
to new barrier and
repeat three to four
times.

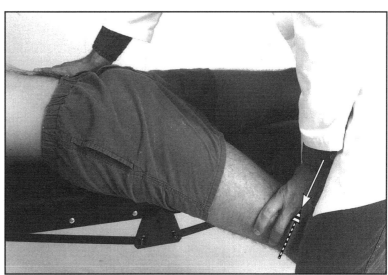

Notes

Direct Operator Assist*   Dx: Innominate Posterior

* Procedure good for treatment of obese patients.

1

Ask patient to stand at arms length from a structure which can be used to balance against.

Ask patient to cross foot on side with somatic dysfunction over (anterior) the other foot.

(All patient's weight must be on uninvolved leg.)

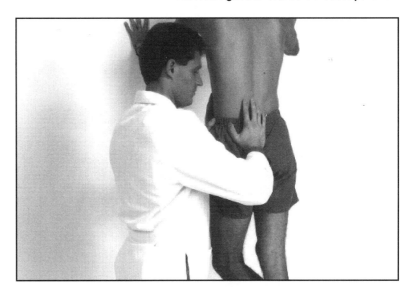

2

Place hands on PSIS and ASIS.

Press anterior superior on PSIS and posterior inferior on ASIS.

Ask patient to lower toward floor while you continue pressure on iliac spine.

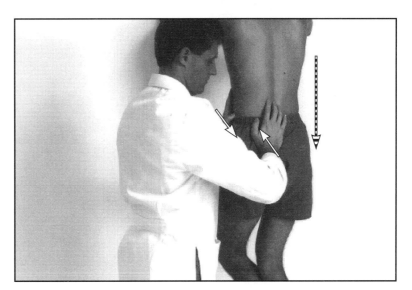

3

As barrier is reached, ask patient to straighten up again.

This procedure may need to be repeated several times.

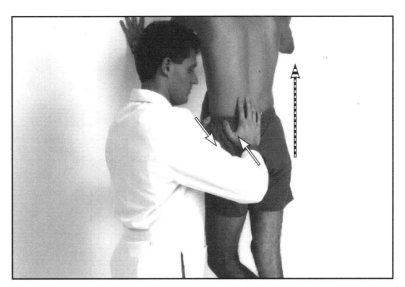

Notes

1

Ask patient to lay on side, with somatic dysfunction up.

Straighten lower leg and flex upper leg.

Place heel of caudal hand on ischial tuberosity and heel of cephlad hand on ASIS.

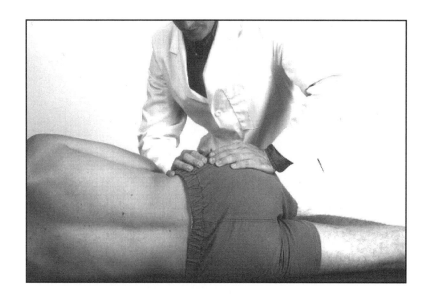

2

Increase tension to barrier and apply short, quick thrust anterior on ischial tuberosity.

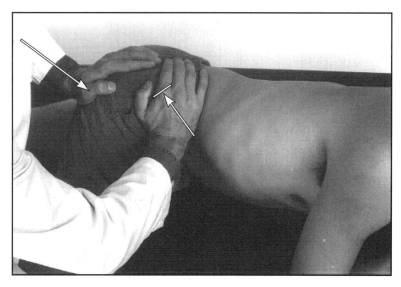

Notes

1

Place forearm on patient's sacrum parallel to vertical axis.

Ask patient to place foot on your knee.

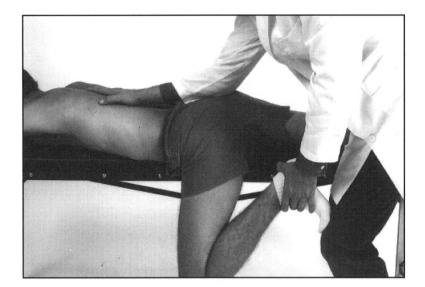

2

Grasp patient's knee with other hand and lean to flex patient's hip.

Carry foot superior to barrier.

Ask patient to press foot against your equally applied force, then relax.

Lift to new barrier again and repeat three to four times.

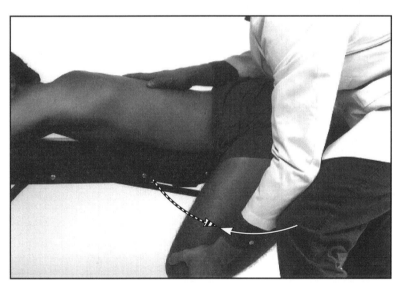

Notes

1 With caudal hand, grasp ischial tuberosity.

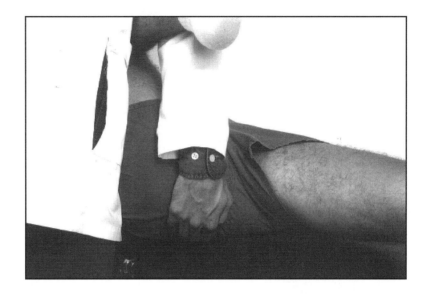

2 Place thenar eminance of cephlad hand against anterior inferior aspect of ASIS.

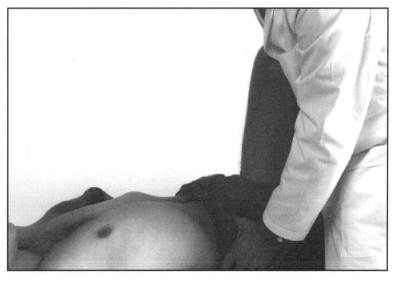

3 Lean on patient's knee to flex and *adduct* the thigh to point of ligamentous tension.

Ask patient to press knee against your equally applied force, then relax.

Flex and *adduct* thigh to new barrier and repeat three to four times.

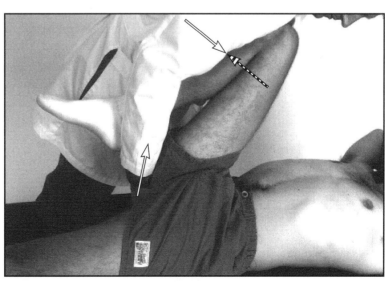

Notes

1

Ask patient to stand at arms length from a structure which can be used to balance against.

Ask patient to cross foot on side with somatic dysfunction over (anterior) the other foot.

(All patient's weight must be on uninvolved leg.)

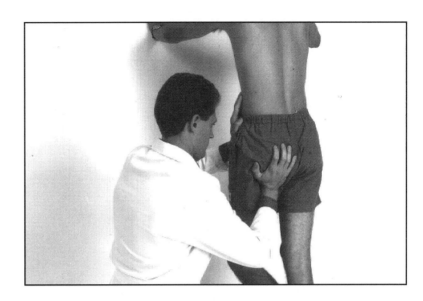

2

Place hands on ASIS and ischial tuberosity.

Press posterior inferior on ASIS and anterior superior on ischial tuberosity.

Ask patient to lower toward floor while you continue pressure on ASIS and ischial tuberosity.

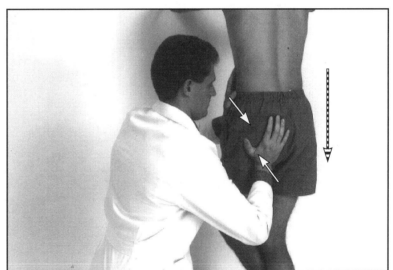

3

As barrier is reached, ask patient to straighten up again.

This procedure may need to be repeated several times.

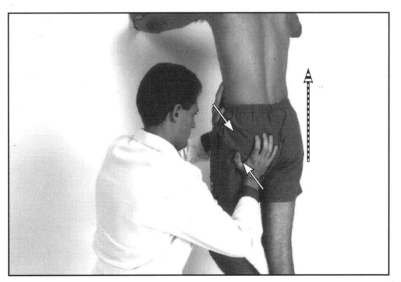

Notes

Direct HVLA   Dx: Sacral Base Anterior

1 Ask patient to slightly flex top leg enough to hang off table.

Support and stabilize patient with forearm against patient's shoulder.

Contact sacrum with other forearm.

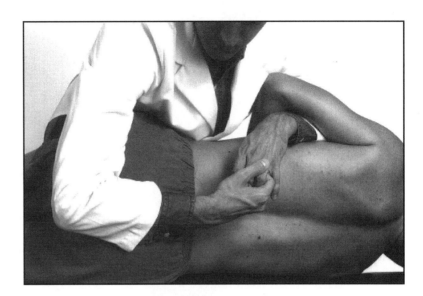

2 Ask patient to rock pelvis backward then forward.

At end of forward rock, increase vector force anterior inferior with the forearm over the sacrum.

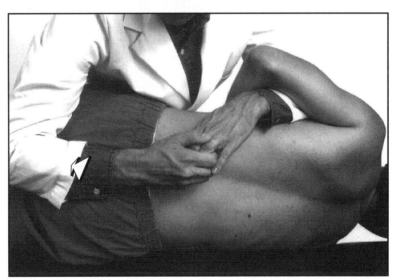

Notes

1   Ask patient to flex knees and raise up to chest.

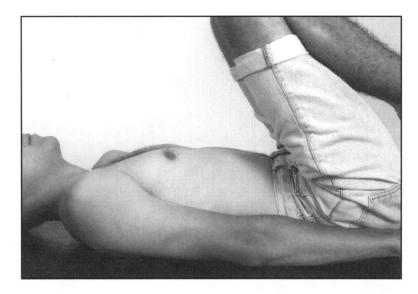

2   Place index and/or middle finger bilaterally to monitor sacral base.

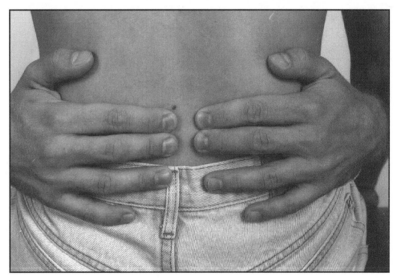

3   Apply pressure on knees to reach barrier.

Ask patient to press knees out against your equally applied force, then relax.

Apply pressure to reach new barrier again and repeat three to four times.

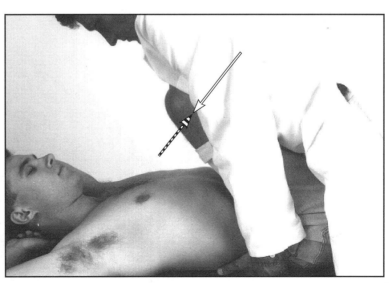

Notes

1 Let sacrum rest in palm of hand.

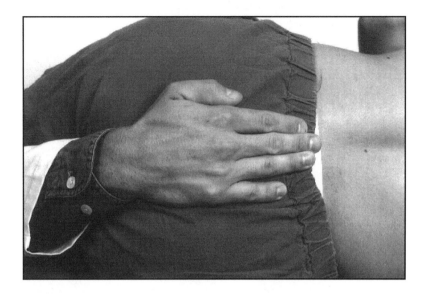

2 Apply pressure with fingers on sacral base to disengage restrictive barrier.

Hold until release is felt.

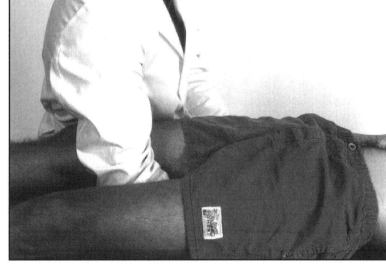

Notes

1 Ask patient to raise up on elbows.

Place heel of one hand on lumbosacral junction.

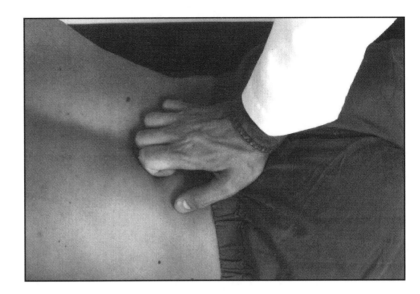

2 Place other hand on lower extremity to stabilize.

Apply pressure on sacral base to reach barrier.

As patient exhales, apply a short, quick thrust anterior.

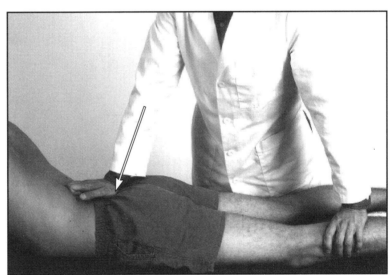

Notes

1 Let sacrum rest in palm of hand.

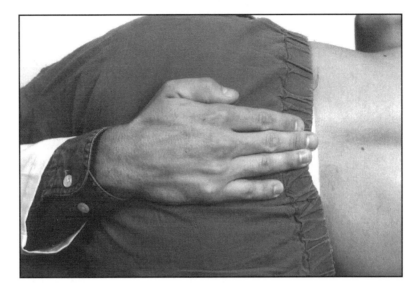

2 Apply pressure with heel of hand on sacral apex to disengage restrictive barrier.

Hold until release is felt.

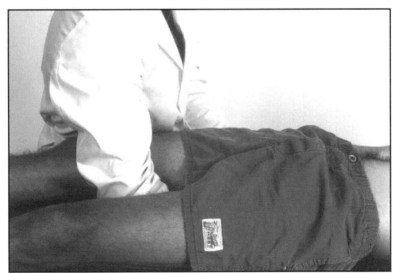

Notes

Direct HVLA   Dx: Sacral Margin Posterior

1

Stand on opposite side of somatic dysfunction.

Pull patient's hip toward you to side-bend around somatic dysfunction.

Ask patient to interlace fingers behind neck.

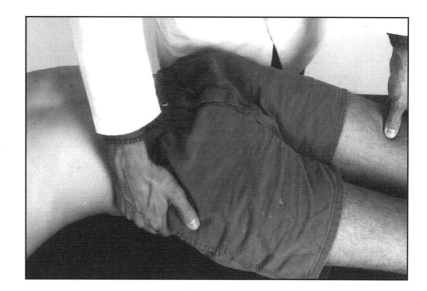

2

Place cephlad hand through patient's opposite arm and rest dorsum of hand on patient's chest.

Place heel of caudal hand on opposite ASIS.

When rotation has occurred down to the sacrum, apply a short, quick thrust against the ASIS.

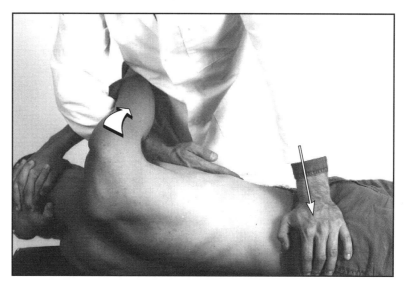

Notes

1

Ask patient to set up arms as shown in photo.

Grasp patient's opposite shoulder or arm.

With other hand, monitor articulation with somatic dysfunction.

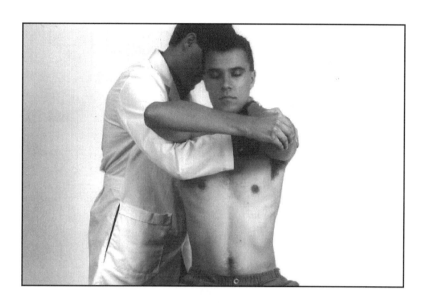

2

Ask patient to sit up straight.

Induce rotation down to barrier.

Ask patient to rotate against your equally applied force, then relax.

Rotate to new barrier again and repeat three to four times.

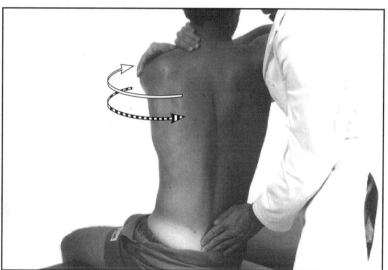

Notes

1 Stand on side with sacrum anterior.

Slide hands under pelvis so fingers of cephlad hand are on sacral base and fingers of caudal hand are on inferior pole of sacro-iliac joint.

Be sure both hands are on margin of sacrum which is anterior.

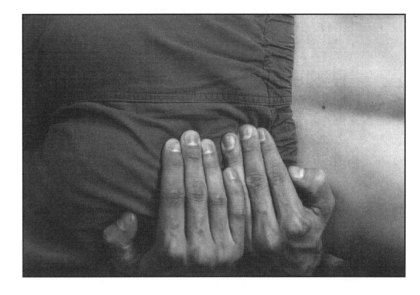

2 Using pressure from both hands, move the sacral margin anterior to disengage the restrictive barrier.

Hold until release is felt.

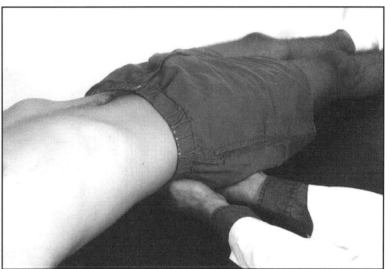

Notes

1

Ask patient to lie prone.

Ask patient to raise right hip and flex hips and knees to 90 degrees or more.

Sit on table and support patient's legs on thigh.

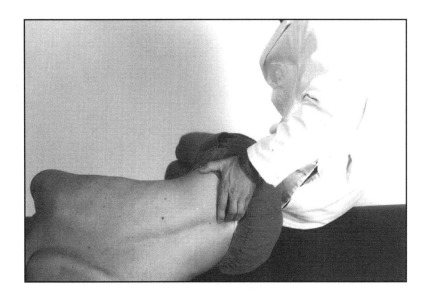

2

Hold patient's ankles and spring two to three times toward floor.

With other hand, grasp spinous process of L-4 and L-5 to induce left rotation.

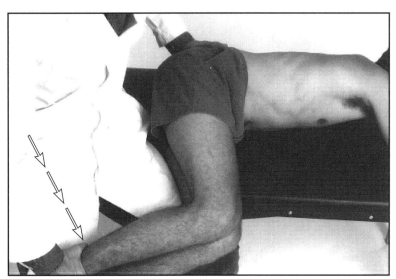

Notes

1

Ask patient to lie prone.

Ask patient to raise right hip and flex hips and knees to 90 degrees or more.

Sit on table and support patient's legs on thigh.

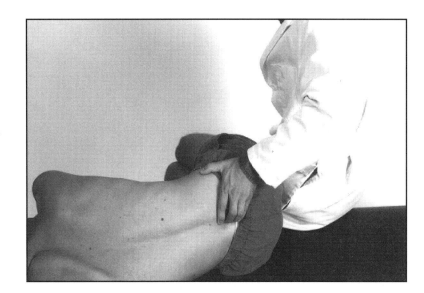

2

Press patient's ankles toward floor until ligamentous tension is felt.

Ask patient to raise ankles toward ceiling against your equally applied force, then relax.

Press ankles toward floor to new barrier and repeat three to four times.

(Use free hand to monitor sacrum during treatment.)

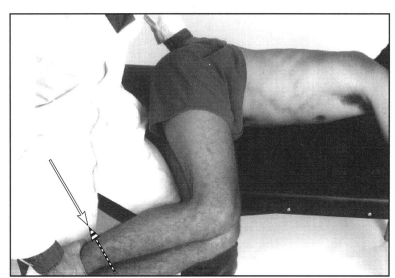

Notes

1 Let sacrum rest in palm of hand.

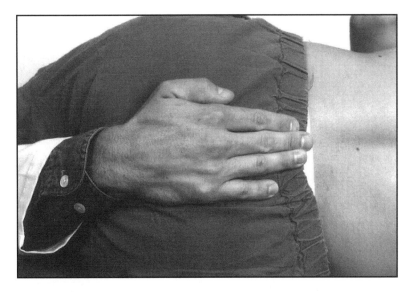

2 Apply pressure with hand to accentuate left oblique axis to disengage restrictive barrier.

(Some tension may be needed in the transverse axis for full release.)

Hold until release is felt.

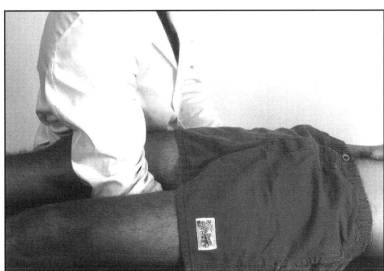

Notes

Direct Springing

1

Stand on patient's left side.

Place hands on right shoulder and on L-5 lumbosacral junction.

Apply gentle springing on right shoulder to induce right rotation.

Use left hand to monitor sacrum during treatment.

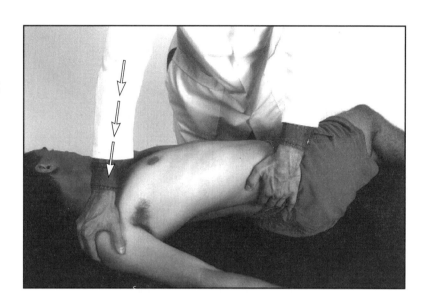

Notes

1 Let sacrum rest in palm of right hand.

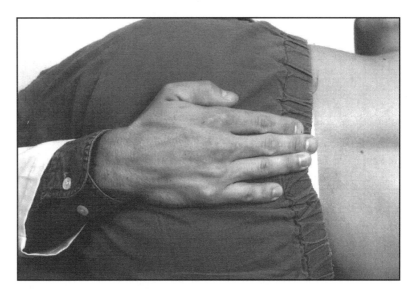

2 Apply pressure with hand to accentuate right rotation on the left oblique axis to disengage restrictive barrier.

Hold until release is felt.

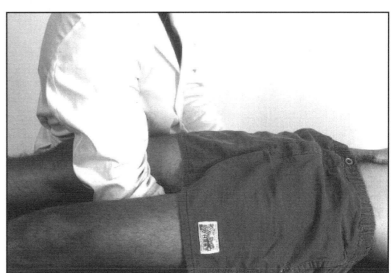

Notes

1 Roll up small hand towel and place under the inferior lateral angle of the sacrum on the inferior shear side.

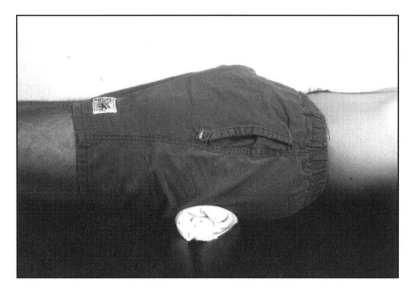

2 Holding patient's ankle, abduct and internally rotate lower extremity.

Ask patient to hold breath.

Apply short, quick tug on leg.

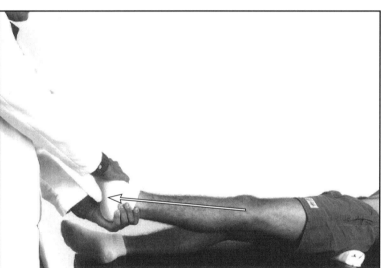

Notes

1 Place thenar eminance on inferior lateral angle of sacrum on side with somatic dysfunction.

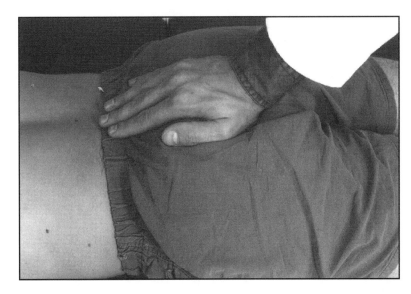

2 Abduct and internally rotate lower extremity.

Ask patient to inhale as you apply increased pressure on sacrum in superior direction.

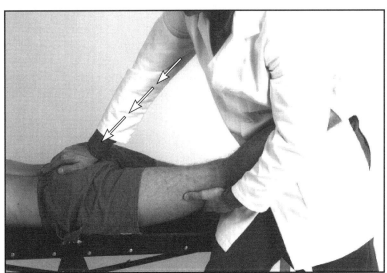

Notes

Direct Springing   Dx: Clavicle Anterior/Superior

1 Place hypothenar eminance on medial one-third of clavicle.

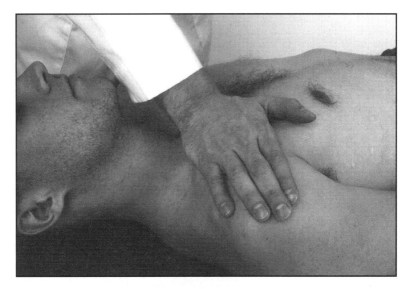

2 Slide caudal forearm between patient's humerus and thorax, high in axilla.

Ask patient to grasp wrist and pull to gap clavicular joints.

Apply spring pressure in a posterior inferior direction on medial clavicle.

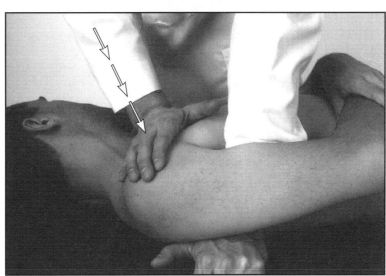

Notes

1

Place thumbs on inferior surface of middle one-third of clavicle.

Monitor sterno-clavicular and acromioclavicular joints with index and middle fingers of each hand.

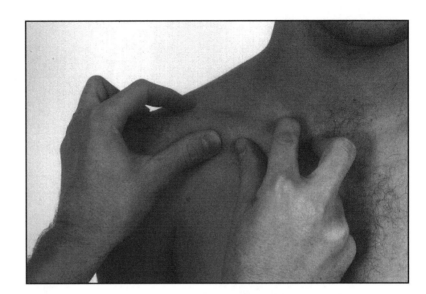

2

Ask patient to lean forward against your thumbs until restrictive barrier is disengaged.

Hold until release is felt.

(Forces should be concentrated to SC joint.)

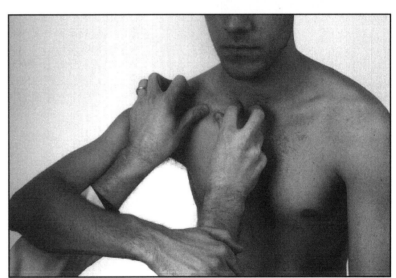

Notes

1 Place thumb on posterior aspect of lateral clavicle.

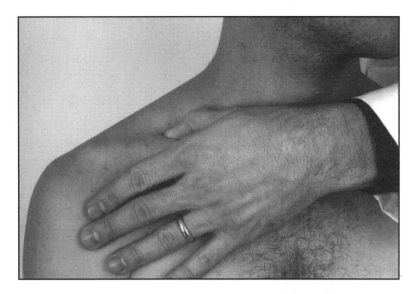

2 Grasp distal humerus.

Extend and adduct to move clavicle anterior.

Press on clavicle with thumb to hold in fixed position.

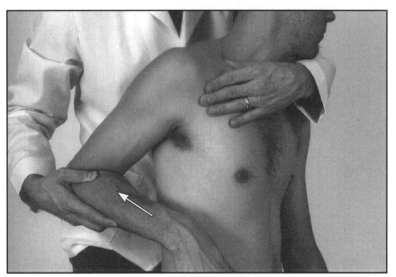

3 Move the humerus into flexion using a quick, whipping motion.

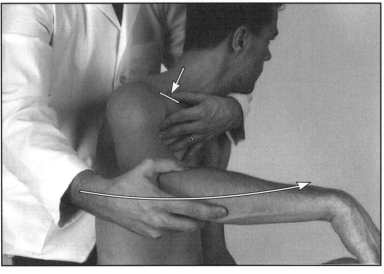

Notes

CLAVICLE—AC

1 Place thumbs on inferior surface of middle one-third of clavicle.

Monitor sterno-clavicular and acromioclavicular joints with index and middle fingers of each hand.

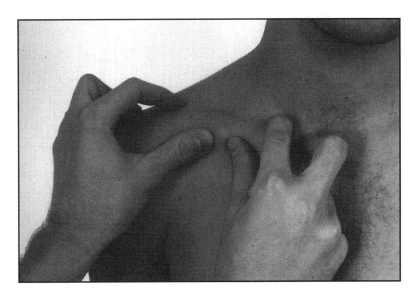

2 Ask patient to lean forward against your thumbs until restrictive barrier is disengaged.

Hold until release is felt.

(Forces should be concentrated to AC joint).

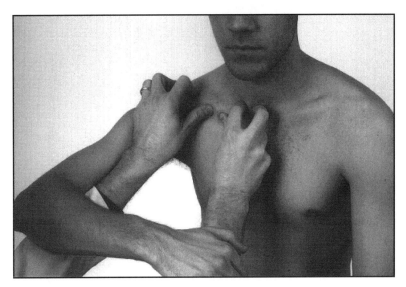

Notes

1 Place web of thumb and index finger over humeral head.

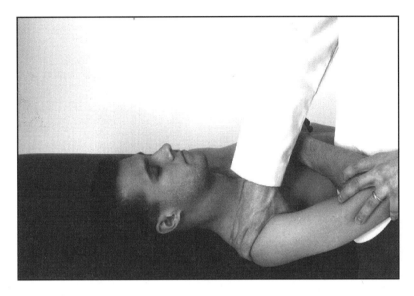

2 Flex, adduct and internally rotate humerus to barrier.

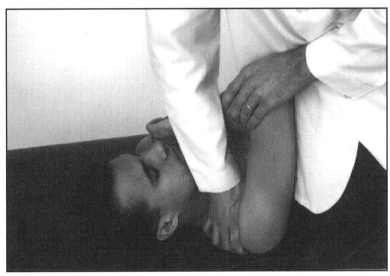

3 Apply a short, quick thrust in a posterior inferior direction.

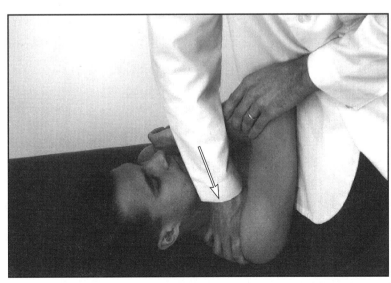

Notes

1 Monitor humeral head with one hand and grasp the upper one-third of the humerus with the other.

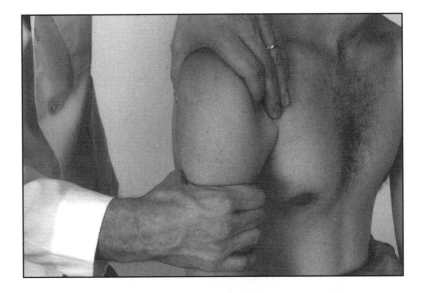

2 Ask patient to grasp his/her elbow and pull arm across chest away from side with somatic dysfunction.

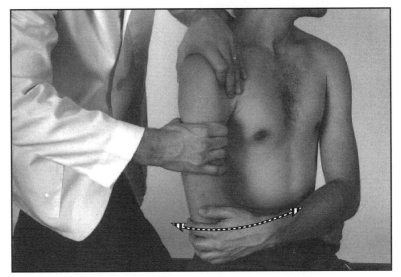

3 Operator and patient may need to adjust accordingly to disengage restrictive barrier.

Hold until release is felt.

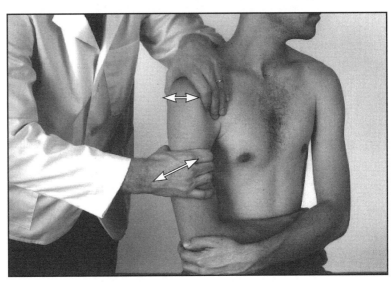

Notes

*(7 Stages of Spencer)

1

Extension (80 to 90°)**:**

Support acromioclavicular joint with one hand to prevent rotation of the scapula.

Test motion in parasagittal plane with other hand, as shown.

If restrictions are noted, use muscle energy techniques three to five times.

Follow up with step 2 (below).

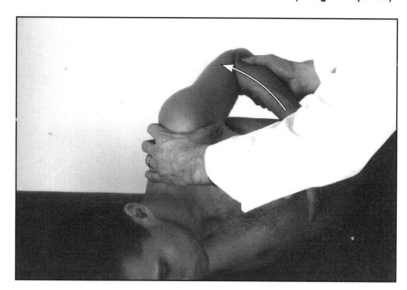

2

Flexion (180°)**:**

Support acromioclavicular joint with one hand.

Test motion in parasagittal plane with other hand, as shown.

If restrictions are noted, use muscle energy techniques three to five times.

Follow up with step 3 (next page).

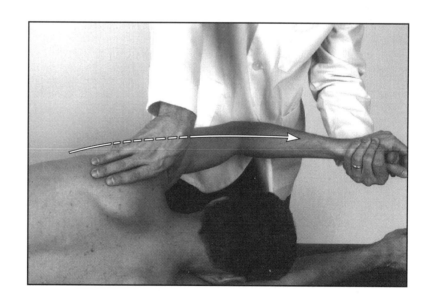

Notes

3

Circumduction with Compression:

Support acromio-clavicular joint with one hand. Cup other hand over patient's elbow. Abduct arm in coronal plane to 90 degrees.

Apply compression and circumduct arm clockwise and then counter-clockwise.

Note areas of resistance. Work through gently by changing circumference and compression.

Follow-up with step 4 (below).

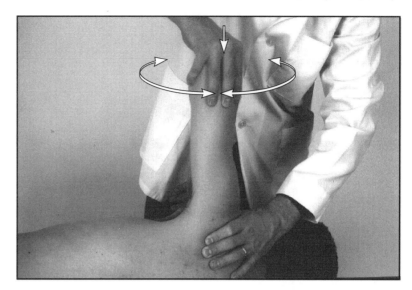

4

Circumduction with Traction:

Support acromio-clavicular joint with one hand.

Flex patient's elbow over web between thumb and index finger of other hand.

Abduct arm in coronal plane to 90°.

Apply traction and circumduct arm clockwise and then counterclockwise.

Work gently through resistance by changing circum-ference and traction.

Follow-up with step 5 (next page).

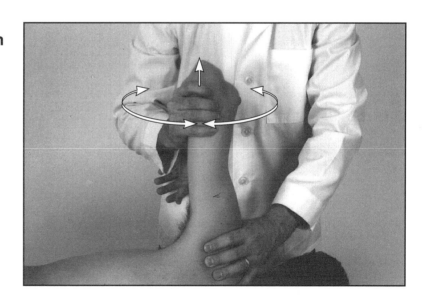

GLENOHUMERAL JOINT

209

Notes

5

Abduction(80-90°):

Support acromioclavicular joint with one hand.

Test motion in coronal plane using other hand as shown.

If restrictions are noted, use muscle energy techniques three to five times.

Follow-up with step 6 (below).

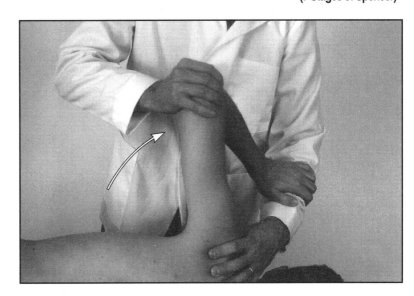

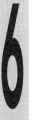

6

Internal Rotation (30°):

Ask patient to place the posterior aspect of hand near PSIS.

Support acromioclavicular joint with one hand.

Grasp patient's elbow and move in anterior direction.

If restrictions are noted, use muscle energy techniques three to five times.

Follow-up with step 7 (next page).

(An external rotation test and treatment may also be added from this position.)

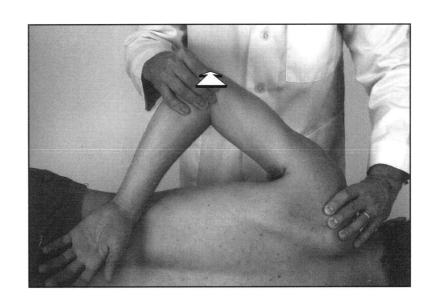

GLENOHUMERAL JOINT

Notes

*(7 Stages of Spencer)

7

Caudal glide (pump) of the Humeral Head:

Extend patient's arm and hand to rest on your shoulder.

Interlock fingers over the humeral head.

Using a pumping action, glide the humeral head caudally and lateral.

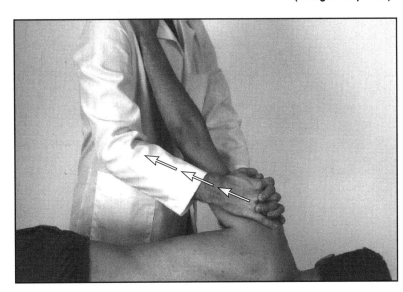

Notes

1 Place thenar eminance on medial proximal aspect of ulna.

Grasp lateral distal aspect of forearm with other hand.

Adduct ulna to barrier.

(Ulno-humeral joint should be just short of full extension.)

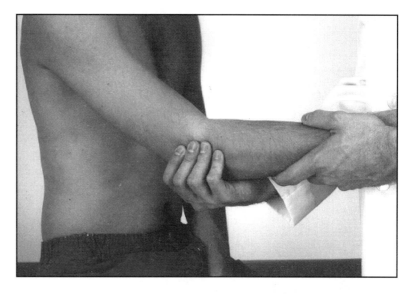

2 While maintaining pressure in adduction, apply a short, quick thrust using both hands simultaneously.

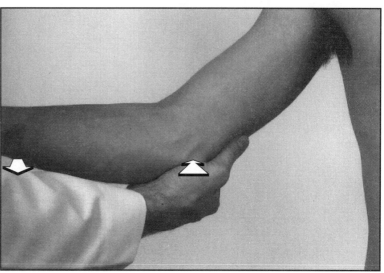

Notes

ULNA

1

Place thenar eminance on medial proximal aspect of ulna.

Grasp lateral distal aspect of forearm with other hand.

Adduct ulna to barrier.

(Ulno-humeral joint should be just short of full extension.)

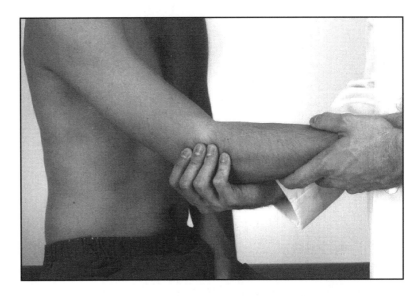

2

While maintaining pressure in adduction, ask patient to abduct forearm against your equally applied force, then relax.

Adduct ulna again to reach new barrier and repeat three to four times.

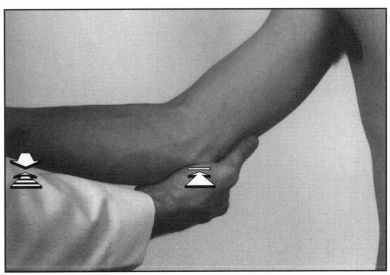

Notes

1

Place thenar eminance on lateral proximal aspect of ulna.

Grasp medial distal aspect of forearm with other hand.

Abduct ulna to barrier.

(Ulno-humeral joint should be just short of full extension.)

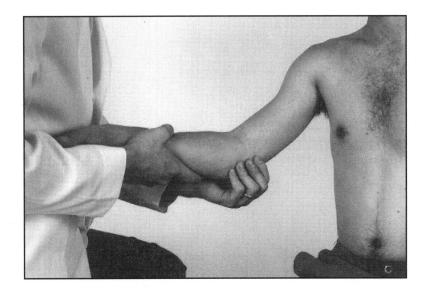

2

While maintaining pressure in abduction, apply a short, quick thrust using both hands simultaneously.

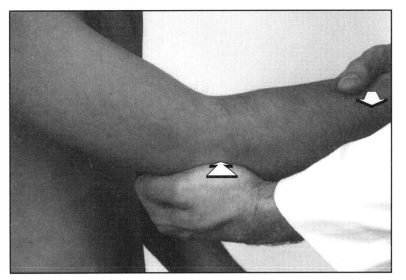

Notes

1

Place thenar eminance on lateral proximal aspect of ulna.

Grasp medial distal aspect of forearm with other hand.

Abduct ulna to barrier.

(Ulno-humeral joint should be just short of full extension.)

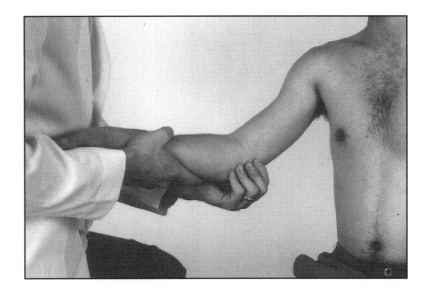

2

While maintaining pressure in abduction, ask patient to adduct forearm against your equally applied force, then relax.

Abduct ulna again to reach new barrier and repeat three to four times.

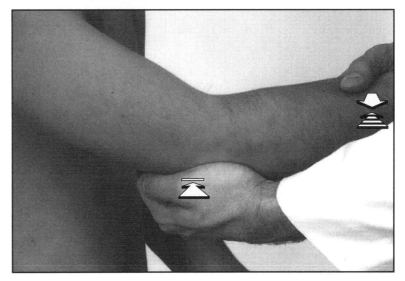

Notes

1

Place index finger and thumb on proximal forearm to monitor radial head.

With other hand, grasp patient's hand in hand-shake fashion.

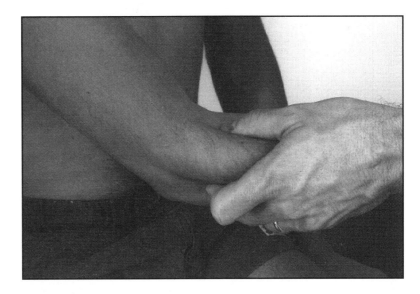

2

Supinate forearm until barrier is reached.

Ask patient to pronate against your equally applied force, then relax.

Supinate again to reach new barrier and repeat three to four times.

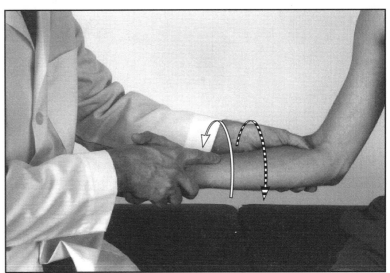

Notes

1 Place hypothenar eminance against proximal radial head in antecubital fossa.

Grasp patient's hand as shown.

Pronate and flex arm until barrier is reached.

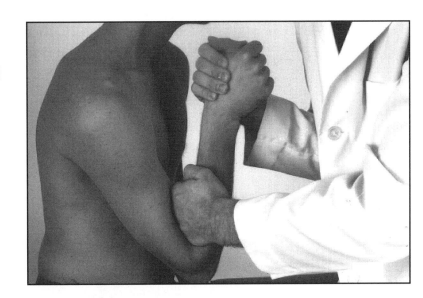

2 Apply a short, quick force to increase flexion.

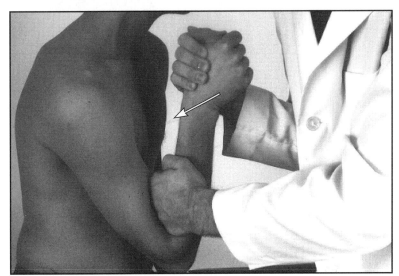

Notes

1

Place index finger and thumb on proximal forearm to monitor radial head.

With other hand, grasp patient's hand in hand-shake fashion.

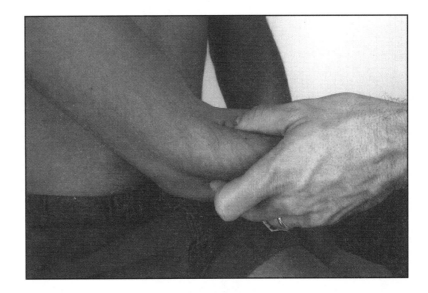

2

Pronate forearm until barrier is reached.

Ask patient to supinate against your equally applied force, then relax.

Pronate again to reach new barrier and repeat three to four times.

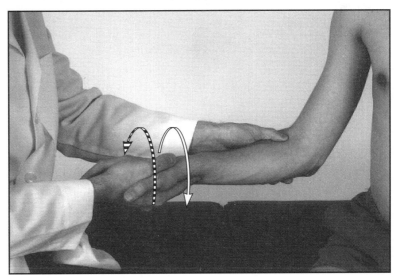

Notes

Direct HVLA

Dx: Flexion

1

Place hands as shown in photo with thumbs over proximal row of carpal bones.

Apply traction to gap joint.

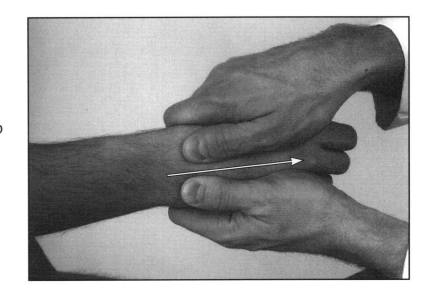

2

Maintain traction while carrying wrist into flexion.

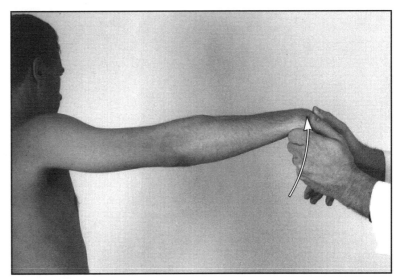

3

Continue to maintain traction and quickly extend wrist through restrictive barrier.

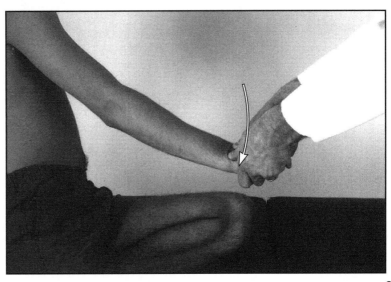

229

Notes

Circumduction

1 Interlace fingers and grasp patient's wrist as shown.

Apply traction to gap joint.

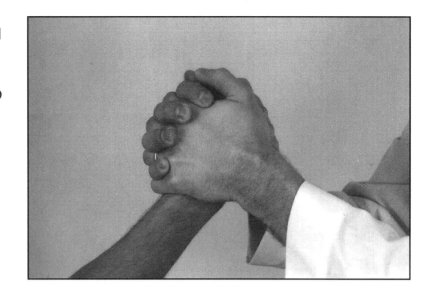

2 Circumduct the wrist, taking it through its range of motion.

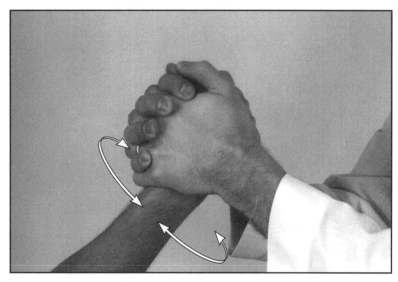

Notes

1 Place hands as shown in photo with thumbs over proximal row of carpal bones.

Apply traction to gap joint.

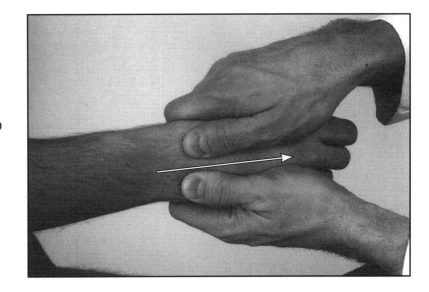

2 Maintain traction while carrying wrist into flexion.

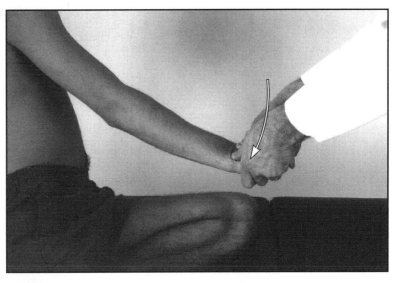

3 Continue to maintain traction and quickly extend wrist through restrictive barrier.

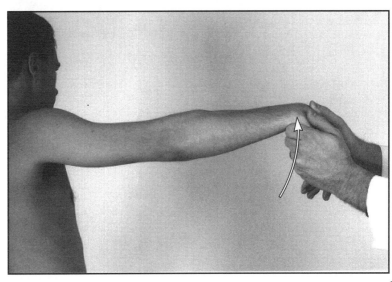

Notes

Circumduction

Dx: Extension

1

Interlace fingers and grasp patient's wrist as shown.

Apply traction to gap joint.

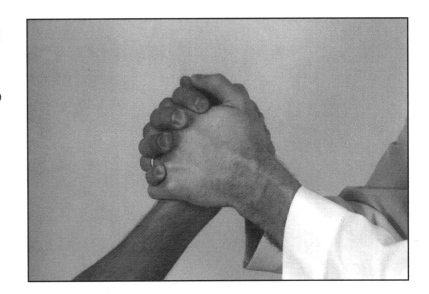

2

Circumduct the wrist, taking it through its range of motion.

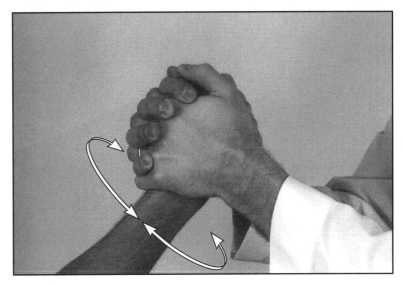

Notes

1 *(NOTE: Correct any somatic dysfunction of the ulna prior to treating abduction of the wrist.)*

Place hands as shown in photo with thumbs near lateral margins of proximal row of carpal bones.

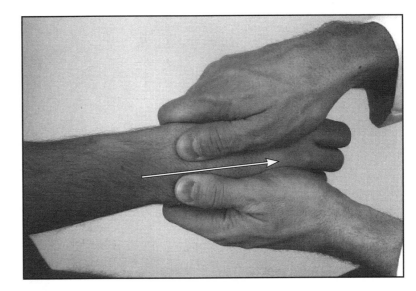

2 Maintain traction while carrying wrist into abduction.

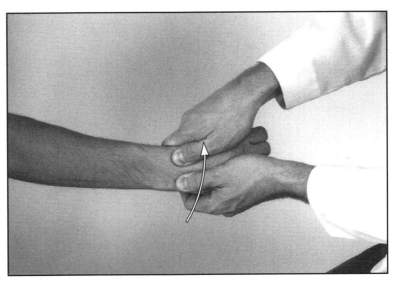

3 While maintaining traction, quickly adduct wrist through restrictive barrier.

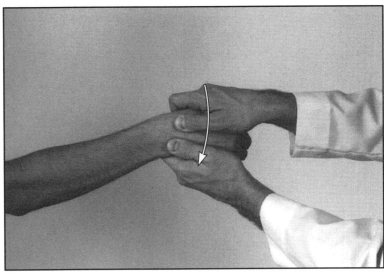

Notes

1 *(NOTE: Correct any somatic dysfunction of the ulna prior to treating adduction of the wrist.)*

Place hands as shown in photo with thumbs near lateral margins of proximal row of carpal bones.

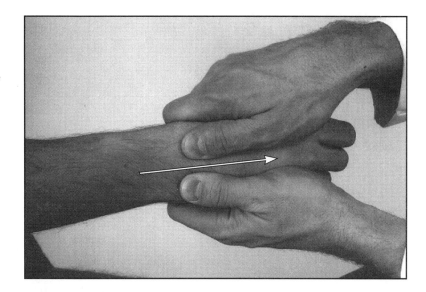

2 Maintain traction while carrying wrist into adduction.

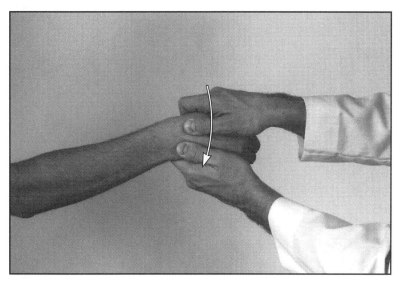

3 While maintaining traction, quickly abduct wrist through restrictive barrier.

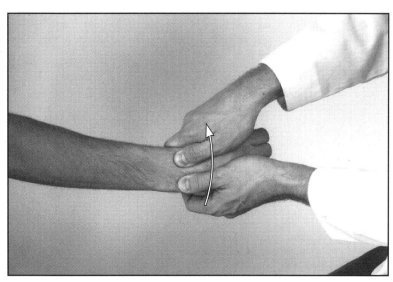

Notes

Somatic dysfunction of intercarpal articulations are similar to wrist articulations such as Flexion, Extension, Abduction, Adduction.

Circumduction procedures are similar to those for the wrist except pressure between the hands of the operator is located over the intercarpal bone.

HVLA procedures are also similar to treatments for the wrist except thumbs are placed over the intercarpal bones with the somatic dysfunction.

Please see pages 229 to 235.

Treatments are similar to HVLA procedures for abduction and adduction of wrist except thumbs are placed in appropriate position over carpal bone with somatic dysfunction.

Please see pages 237 and 239.

Notes

Direct HVLA

1

Place hands as shown in photo.

Apply traction to restrictive barrier.

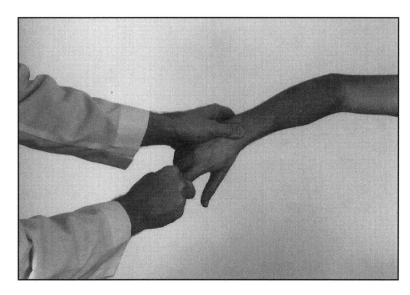

2

Apply short, quick pull distally as shown in photo.

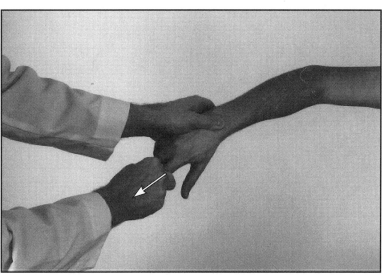

Notes

1

Grasp patient's finger as shown.

Glide joint to disengage restrictive barrier.

Hold until release is felt.

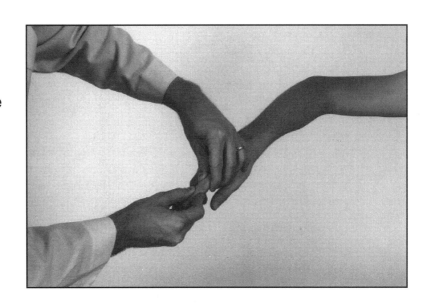

METACARPAL PHALANGEAL ARTICULATION

Notes

1

Grasp patient's finger as shown.

Glide joint to disengage restrictive barrier.

Hold until release is felt.

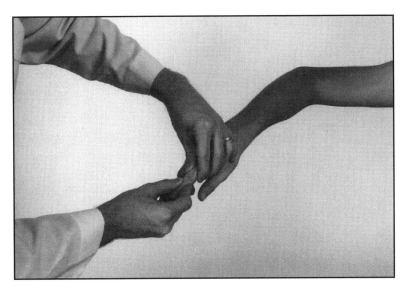

Notes

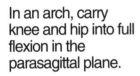

Flex knee and hip.

Carry thigh into adduction and internally rotate to disengage restrictive barrier.

Ask patient to externally rotate entire lower extremity against your equally applied force, then relax.

Repeat three to four times.

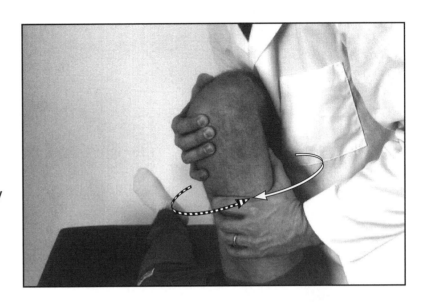

In an arch, carry knee and hip into full flexion in the parasagittal plane.

Ask patient to extend knee and hip against your equally applied force, then relax.

Apply pressure to flex knee and hip to point of ligamentous tension.

Repeat three to four times.

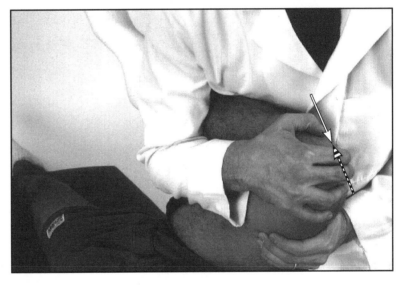

In an arch, carry knee into abduction and externally rotate until barrier is reached.

Ask patient to internally rotate against your equally applied force, then relax.

Externally rotate to new barrier again and repeat three to four times.

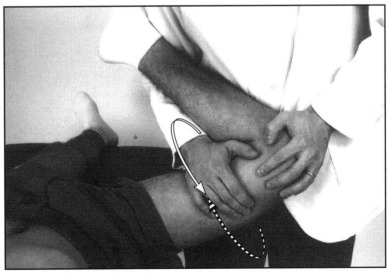

Notes

1

Grasp patient's distal calf with caudad hand.

Flex knee and hip, and externally rotate thigh to point of tension.

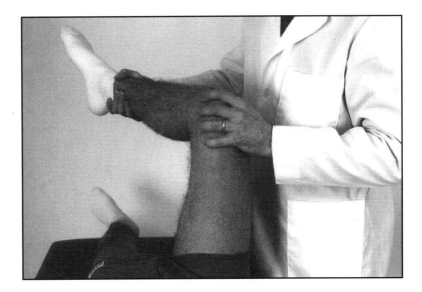

2

Ask patient to internally rotate entire lower extremity against your equally applied force, then relax.

Externally rotate to new barrier again and repeat three to four times.

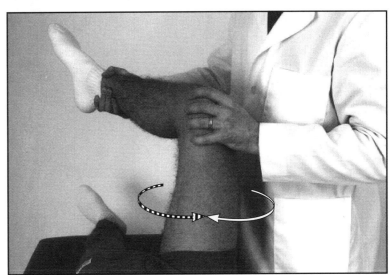

Notes

1 Place hand on medial proximal aspect of femur to act as a fulcrum.

Ask patient to cross the leg on the involved side.

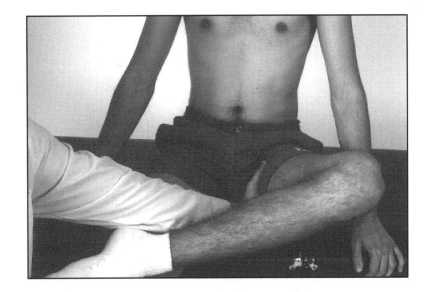

2 Place other hand on patient's knee and lift or lower knee to position of least hip tension.

Ask patient to cross legs and lean forward and toward side with somatic dysfunction (photo).

Place your other hand on patient's knee.

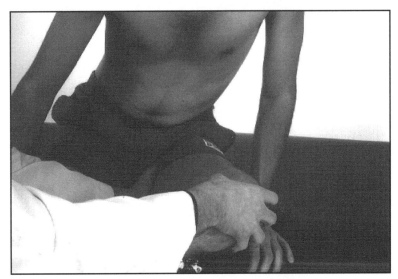

3 Lift or lower knee to disengage restrictive barrier.

Hold until release is felt.

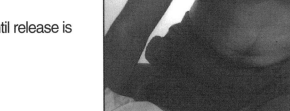
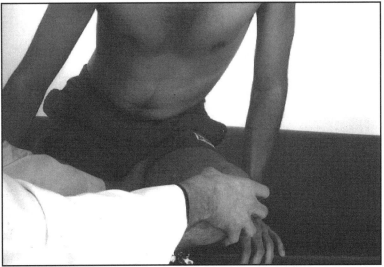

Notes

1

Flex knee and hip.

Carry thigh into abduction and externally rotate to disengage restrictive barrier.

Ask patient to internally rotate entire lower extremity against your equally applied force, then relax.

Repeat three to four times.

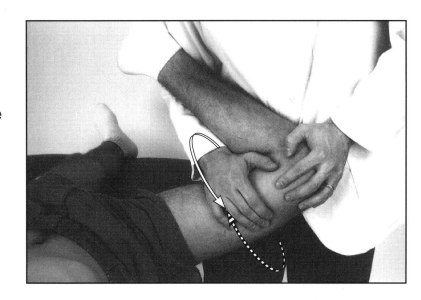

2

In an arch, carry knee and hip into full flexion in the parasagittal plane.

Ask patient to extend knee and hip against your equally applied force, then relax.

Apply pressure to flex knee and hip to point of ligamentous tension.

Repeat three to four times.

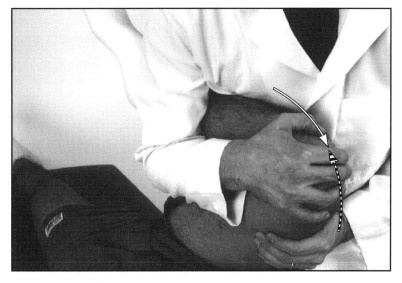

3

In an arch, carry knee into adduction and internally rotate until barrier is reached.

Ask patient to externally rotate against your equally applied force, then relax.

Internally rotate to new barrier again and repeat three to four times.

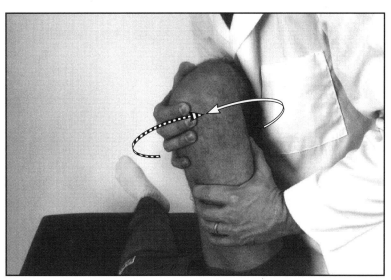

Notes

1

Caution is advised if patient has history of knee problems.

Flex patient's knee and hip to 90 degrees.

Support patient's calf between your elbow and rib cage.

Grasp knee and thigh (photo).

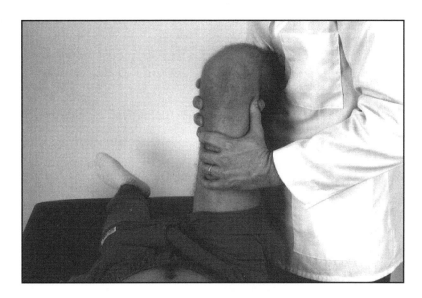

2

Internally rotate thigh to point of tension.

Ask patient to externally rotate against your equally applied force, then relax.

Internally rotate to new barrier again and repeat three to four times.

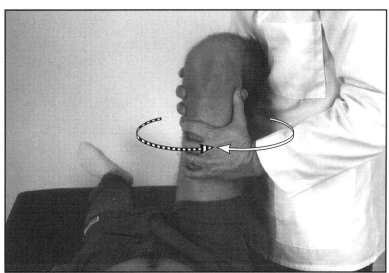

Notes

1

Place hands under posterior aspect of femoral head for monitoring.

Ask patient to cross legs and lean backward and away from side with somatic dysfunction (photo).

Lift or lower patient's knee to disengage restrictive barrier.

Hold until release is felt.

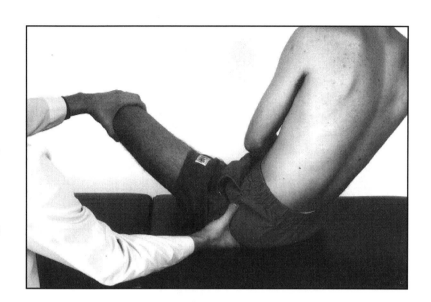

Notes

1

Extend and support patient's lower extremity (photo).

Flex at hip to point of tension.

Ask patient to pull heel toward the buttocks against your equally applied force, then relax.

Flex to new barrier again and repeat three to four times.

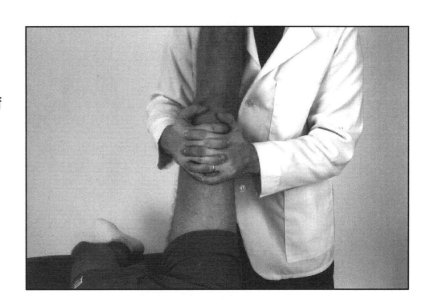

Notes

1

Support patient's knee with small pillow.

Place one hand on distal posterior aspect of femur.

Place heel of other hand on anterior tibia.

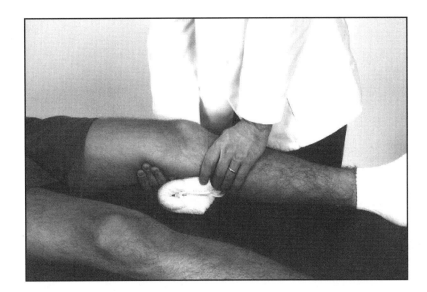

2

Lift femur while applying a short, quick posterior thrust on tibia.

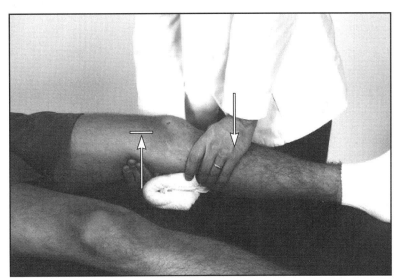

Notes

1 Support patient's knee with small pillow.

Place hands on distal anterior aspect of femur.

Grasp medial posterior aspect of tibial head.

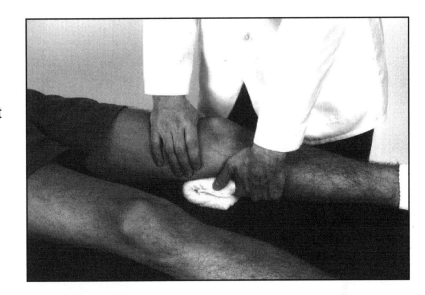

2 Lift tibia while applying a short, quick posterior thrust on femur.

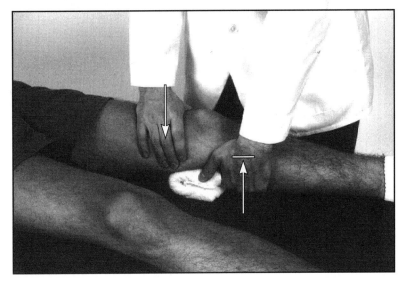

Notes

1

Place cephlad hand against lateral condyle of tibia.

Support ankle with other hand.

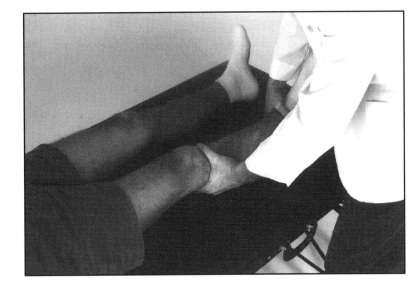

2

Apply a springing motion medial on tibial condyle while pulling ankle lateral.

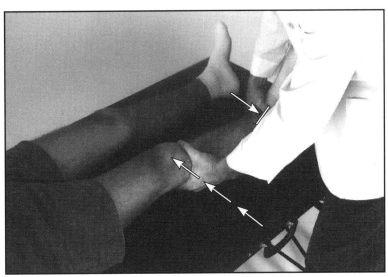

Notes

1 Place cephlad hand against medial condyle of tibia.

Support ankle with other hand.

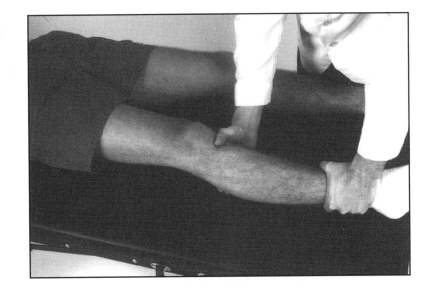

2 Apply lateral springing motion on tibial condyle while pulling ankle medial.

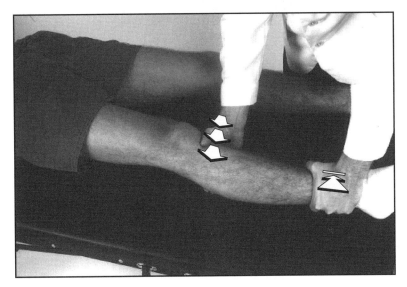

Notes

1

Ask patient to sit with legs hanging off edge of table.

Monitor tibial plateau with thumb and index finger.

Grasp patient's ankle and apply downward traction with other hand.

Internally or externally rotate tibia to disengage restrictive barrier.

Hold until release is felt.

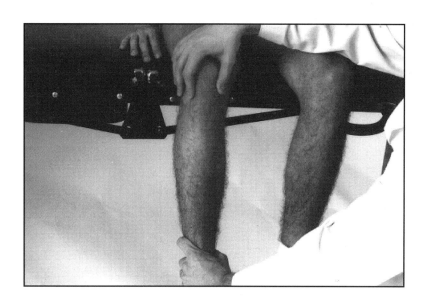

Notes

1

Ask patient to sit with legs hanging off edge of table.

Monitor tibial plateau with thumb and index finger.

Grasp patient's ankle and apply downward traction with other hand.

Internally or externally rotate tibia to disengage restrictive barrier.

Hold until release is felt.

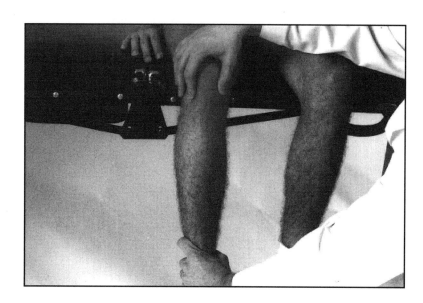

Notes

1

Place hands as shown in photo, with thumb against posterior aspect of proximal fibular head.

Flex knee and hip, and externally rotate tibia until tension develops at proximal fibular head.

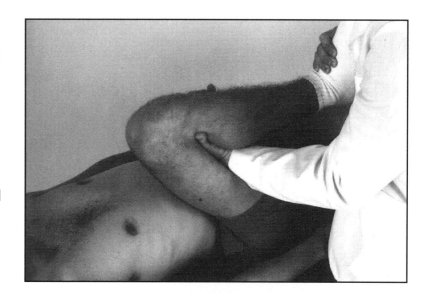

2

Evert and dorsiflex the foot to increase tension at proximal fibular head.

Apply a short, quick thrust, accentuating the knee flexion, tibial rotation, eversion and dorsiflexion simultaneously.

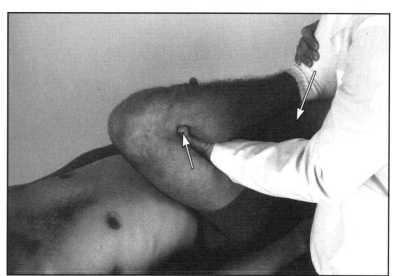

Notes

1 Suspend patient's leg by grasping fibular head and lateral malleolus between thumb and index finger (photo).

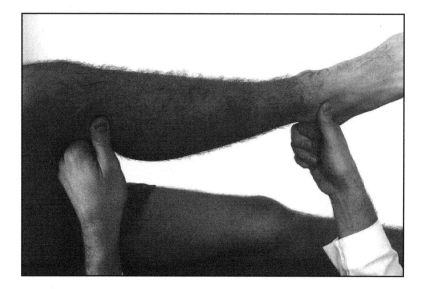

2 Glide fibular head and lateral malleolus to point of disengaging restrictive barrier.

Hold until release is felt.

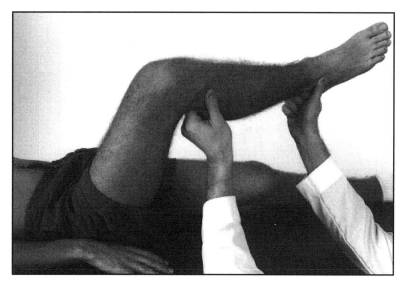

Notes

1 Suspend patient's leg by grasping fibular head and lateral malleolus between thumb and index finger (photo).

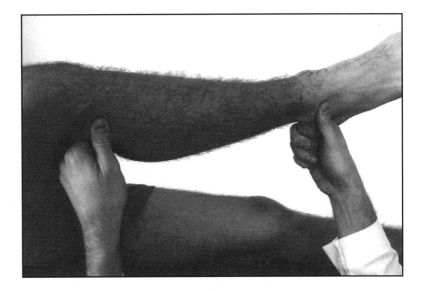

2 Glide fibular head and lateral malleolus to point of disengaging restrictive barrier.

Hold until release is felt.

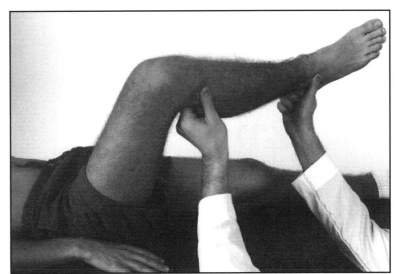

Notes

1   Grasp patient's foot by interlacing fingers around head of talus (photo).

Dorsiflex ankle to barrier and maintain that tension.

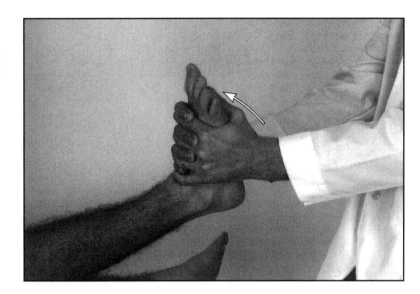

2   Apply a short, quick pull in a caudal direction.

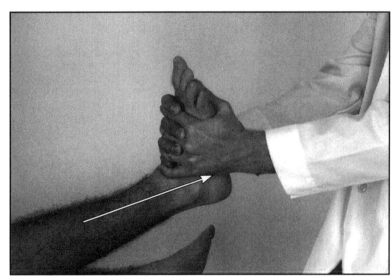

Notes

Dx: Talus Plantar Flexed

1

Support patient's leg (photo).

Using thumb and index finger, apply caudal force to heel.

With other hand grasp ball of foot and apply cephlad force to dorsiflex foot.

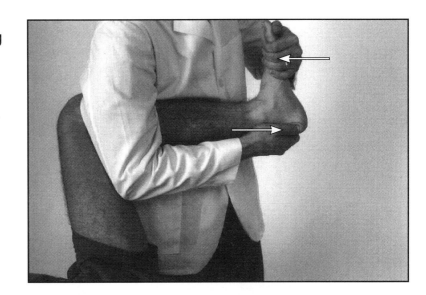

2

Ask patient to plantar flex against your equal force, then relax.

Dorsiflex to new barrier again and repeat three to four times.

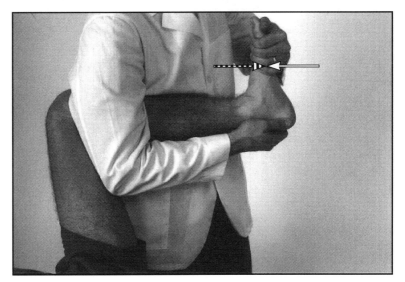

Notes

1

Grasp heel with palm of hand.

With other hand, press hypothenar eminance against head of talus on medial side of foot.

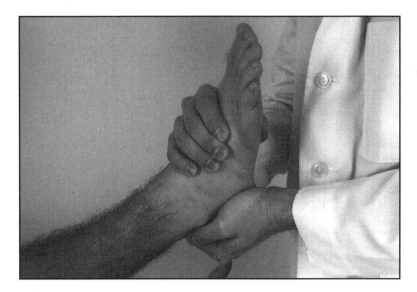

2

Apply a short, quick thrust against the talar head posterolaterally while thrusting the calcaneous medial.

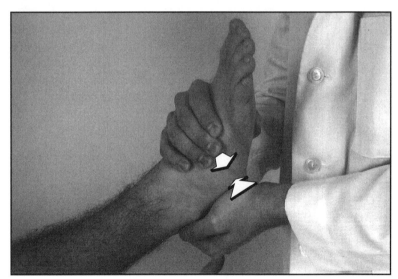

Notes

1

Grasp heel with palm of hand.

Apply traction in a caudal direction.

Use thumb and index finger on talar head to monitor and move talus to disengage restrictive barrier.

Hold until release is felt.

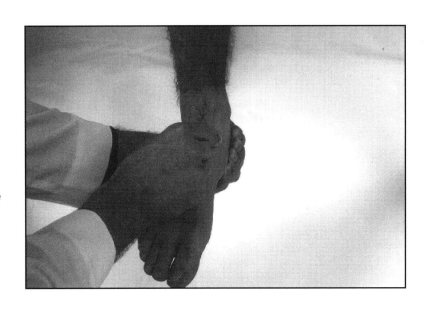

Notes

1 Grasp heel with palm of hand.

With other hand, press hypothenar eminance against head of talus on lateral side of foot.

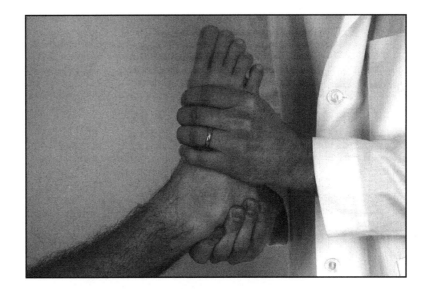

2 Apply a short, quick thrust against the talar head anteromedially while thrusting calcaneous lateral.

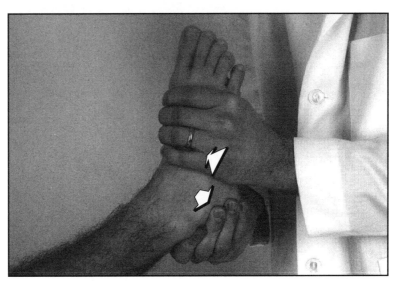

Notes

1

Grasp heel with palm of hand.

Apply traction in a caudal direction.

Use thumb and index finger on talar head to monitor and move talus to disengage restrictive barrier.

Hold until release is felt.

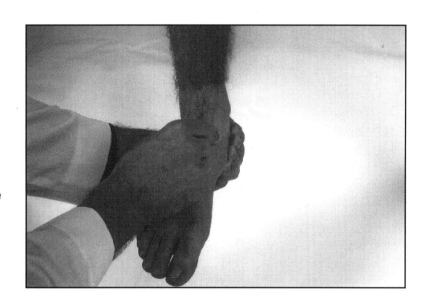

Notes

1

Grasp foot (photo).

Place thumb in contact with cuboid.

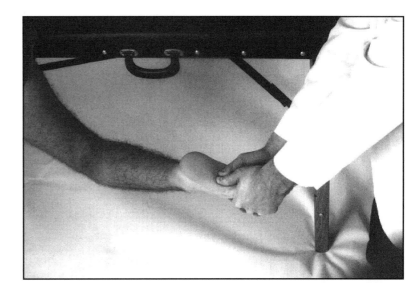

2

Carry foot medial to lateral and apply a short, quick thrust as lateral barrier is reached.

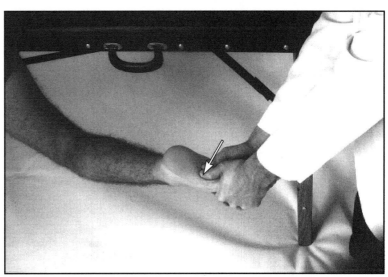

Notes

1 Grasp foot (photo).

Place thumb in contact with cuneiform.

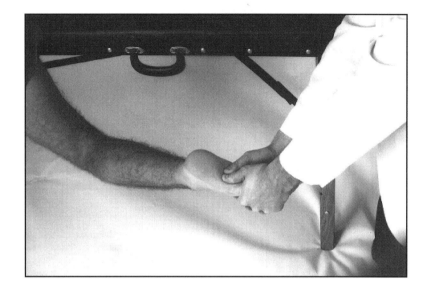

2 Carry foot medial to lateral.

At half way point between medial and lateral barriers, apply a short, quick thrust downward.

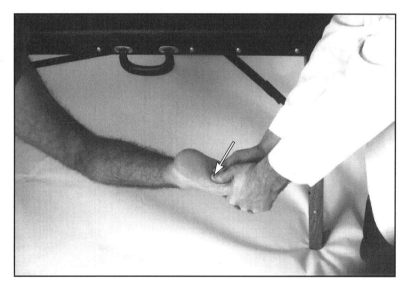

Notes

1

Grasp foot (photo).

Place thumb in contact with navicular.

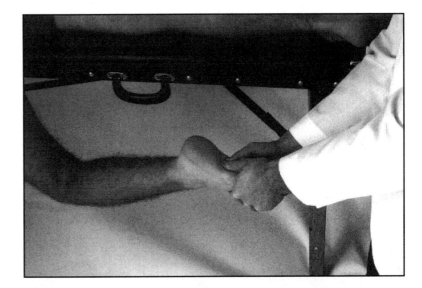

2

Carry foot from lateral to medial and apply a short, quick thrust as medial barrier is reached.

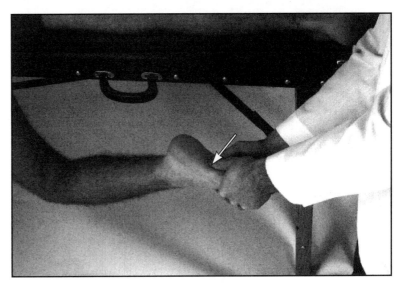

AA JOINT
Dx: RR
    Direct ME 17
    Indirect 19

ANKLE
Dx: Talus Plantar Flexed
    Direct HVLA 281
    Direct ME 283

CERVICAL C2-C6
Dx: BB
    Direct ME 27
    Indirect 29
Dx: FB
    Direct HVLA 21
    Direct ME 23
    Indirect 25
Dx: N $S_R R_R$
    Direct HVLA (Side-bending) 31
    Direct ME 33
    Indirect 35
Dx: NN $S_R R_R$ (Rare)
    Please refer to page 37.

CLAVICLE— SC
Dx: Clavicle Anterior/Superior
    Direct Springing 195
    Indirect 197

CLAVICLE— AC
Dx: Clavicle Anterior/Superior
    Direct HVLA 199
    Indirect 201

FIBULA
Dx: Fibular Head Anterior
    Indirect 279
Dx: Fibular Head Posterior
    Direct HVLA 275
    Indirect 277

FOOT
Dx: Cuboid Eversion
    Direct HVLA 293
Dx: Cuneiform Depression
    Direct HVLA 295
Dx: Navicular Inversion
    Direct HVLA 297
Dx: Talus Anteromedial
    Direct HVLA 285
    Indirect 287
Dx: Talus Posterolateral
    Direct HVLA 289
    Indirect 291

HAND
Intercarpal Articulations
    Please refer to page 241.
Carpal Metacarpal Articulation
    Direct HVLA 243
Interphalangeal Articulation
  Dx: Glide Somatic Dysfunction
    Indirect 247
Metacarpal Phalangeal Articulation
  Dx: Glide Somatic Dysfunction
    Indirect 245

HIP
Dx: Internal Rotation
    Direct ME 251
    Indirect 253
    Indirect/Direct Combined 249
Dx: External Rotation
    Direct ME 257
    Indirect 259
    Indirect/Direct Combined 255

KNEE
Dx: Tibia Anterior
    Direct HVLA 263
Dx: Tibia Anteromedial
    Indirect 271
Dx: Tibia Lateral
    Direct Springing 267
Dx: Tibia Medial
    Direct Springing 269
Dx: Tibia Posterior
    Direct HVLA 265
Dx: Tibia Posterolateral
    Indirect 273

LUMBAR T11-L5
Dx: BB
    Direct HVLA 121
    Direct ME 123
    Indirect 125
Dx: FB
    Direct HVLA 117
    Direct ME 119
Dx: N $S_R R_L$
    Direct HVLA 127
    Direct ME 129
    Indirect 131
Dx: NN $R_L S_L$
    Direct HVLA 133
    Direct ME 135
    Indirect 137

OA JOINT
Dx: BB
    Direct ME 7
    Indirect 9
Dx: FB
    Direct HVLA 1
    Direct ME 3
    Indirect 5
Dx: N $S_R R_L$
    Direct HVLA 11
    Direct ME 13
    Indirect 15

PELVIS
Dx: Innominate Anterior
    Direct HVLA 157
    Direct ME 159
    Direct ME 161
    Direct ME 163
Dx: Innominate Posterior
    Direct HVLA 149
    Direct ME 151
    Direct ME 153
    Direct Operator Assist 155

Dx: Pubic Compression
Direct ME 147
Dx: Symphysis Inferior
Direct ME 143
Indirect 145
Dx: Symphysis Superior
Direct ME 139
Indirect 141

RADIUS
Dx: Radial Head Anterior
Direct HVLA 225
Direct ME 227
Dx: Radial Head Posterior
Direct ME 223

RIB 1
Dx: Depressed Rib 1
Direct ME 113
Indirect 115
Dx: Elevated Rib 1
Direct HVLA 107
Direct ME 109
Indirect 111

RIBS 2-10
Dx: Exhalation
Direct HVLA 93
Direct ME 95
Direct ME 99
Indirect 97
Indirect 101
Dx: Inhalation
Direct HVLA 83
Direct ME 89
Direct Respiratory 85
Indirect 87
Indirect 91

RIBS 11, 12
Dx: Exhalation
Direct ME 105
Dx: Inhalation
Direct ME 103

SACRUM
Dx: R_L on LOA
Direct ME 183
Direct Springing 181
Indirect 185
Dx: R_R on LOA
Direct Springing 187
Indirect 189
Dx: Sacral Base Anterior
Direct HVLA 165
Direct ME 167
Indirect 169
Dx: Sacral Base Posterior
Direct HVLA 171
Indirect 173
Dx: Sacral Margin Posterior
Direct HVLA 175
Direct ME 177
Indirect 179
Dx: Unilateral Sacral Shear
Direct HVLA 191
Direct Springing 193

SHOULDER
Dx: Humeral Head Anterior/Superior
Direct HVLA 203
Indirect 205
Dx: Muscular Restrictions
Motions of Shoulder Joint 207

THIGH
Dx: Short Hamstrings
Direct ME 261

THORACIC, LOWER T4-T10
Dx: BB
Direct HVLA 65
Direct ME 67
Indirect 69
Dx: FB
Direct HVLA 59
Direct HVLA 61
Direct Springing 63
Dx: N S_L R_R
Direct HVLA 71
Direct ME 73
Indirect 75
Dx: NN R_R S_R
Direct HVLA 77
Direct ME 79
Indirect 81

THORACIC, UPPER C7-T3
Dx: BB (Rare)
Direct HVLA 45
Direct ME 47
Indirect 49
Dx: FB
Direct Springing 39
Direct Springing 41
Indirect 43
Dx: N S_R R_L
Direct HVLA 51
Direct ME 53
Indirect 55
Dx: NN R_L S_L or R_R S_R
Please refer to page 57.

ULNA
Dx: Abduction of Ulna
Direct HVLA 215
Direct ME 217
Dx: Adduction of Ulna
Direct HVLA 219
Direct ME 221

WRIST
Dx: Abduction
Direct HVLA 237
Dx: Adduction
Direct HVLA 239
Dx: Extension
Circumduction 235
Direct HVLA 233
Dx: Flexion
Circumduction 231
Direct HVLA 229